TRAUMA, REPETITION, AND AFFECT REGULATION: THE WORK OF PAUL RUSSELL

TRAUMA, REPETITION, AND AFFECT REGULATION: THE WORK OF PAUL RUSSELL

EDITED BY

Judith Guss Teicholz, Ed.D.

AND

Daniel Kriegman, Ph.D.

IN COLLABORATION WITH

Susan Fairfield

WITH CONTRIBUTIONS FROM

E. Virginia Demos

George G. Fishman

Jane H. Leavy

Stephen A. Mitchell

Arnold H. Modell

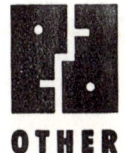

THE OTHER PRESS, LLC
New York

Production Editor: Robert D. Hack

This book was set in 11½ pt. Adobe Caslon by Alpha Graphics of Pittsfield, NH.

Copyright © 1998 by Judith Guss Teicholz and Daniel Kriegman. Chapters 1 and 2 copyright © by Deborah Russell.

All rights reserved, including the right to reproduce this book, or parts thereof, in any form, without written permission from The Other Press, Llc except in the case of brief quotations in reviews for inclusion in a magazine, newspaper, or broadcast. Printed in the United States of America on acid-free paper. For information write to The Other Press, Llc, 377 W. 11th Street, New York, NY 10014. Or visit our website—www.otherpress.com.

Library of Congress Cataloging-in-Publication Data

Trauma, repetition, and affect regulation / edited by Judith Guss
  Teicholz and Daniel Kriegman, in collaboration with Susan Fairfield;
  with contributions from E. Virginia Demos ... [et al.].
      p. cm.
  Includes bibliographical references and index.
  ISBN 1-892746-00-X (softcover : alk. paper)
    1. Repetition compulsion. 2. Psychic trauma. 3. Affect
(Psychology) 4. Psychotherapist and patient. 5. Russell, Paul L.,
M.D. I. Teicholz, Judith Guss. II. Kriegman, Daniel H., 1951-   .
III. Fairfield, Susan.
RC455.4.R42T73 1998
616.85'84—dc21
                                                                    98-36921

CONTENTS

Preface		vii
Contributors		ix
1	The Role of Paradox in the Repetition Compulsion *Paul L. Russell*	1
2	Trauma and the Cognitive Function of Affects *Paul L. Russell*	23
3	Letting the Paradox Teach Us *Stephen A. Mitchell*	49
4	Windows Opened and Closed: Repetition and Deficit in the Negotiation of Affect *Arnold H. Modell*	59
5	Differentiating the Repetition Compulsion from Trauma through the Lens of Tomkins's Script Theory: A Response to Russell *E. Virginia Demos*	67
6	Paradox and the Cognitive Function of Affect: A Discussion of Russell's Papers *George G. Fishman*	105
7	Understanding Repetition and the Treatment Crisis: A View of Paul Russell's Theoretical Orientation *Jane H. Leavy*	123
Index		147

A REMEMBRANCE

Just a few months before he died, I met Paul Russell at a conference where he was the discussant of a paper by a well-known analyst. Paul spoke his mind and minced no words. The audience was somewhat shocked at the directness with which he criticized a viewpoint he felt was seriously flawed. We were accustomed to analytic confrontations that were couched in indirect and veiled presentations. Afterward at lunch with Paul and his wife, Deborah, I asked them about the tone of his discussion, a tone that was, in fact, markedly different from his usual style. It was intentional and Paul was fully aware of how he was coming across. He said he was tired of holding back. There was a certain excitement that Deborah and Paul were sharing about this change in attitude. I think I was witnessing something indicating that a real change was taking place, the kind we see when people go through a major life transition. For me, this added another dimension to the tragic news that came shortly thereafter that Paul had been stricken with the illness that eventually took his life.

Like many psychotherapists around Boston (and beyond), Paul Russell touched my life both directly and indirectly in many ways. I am glad I had the opportunity to help Judy Teicholz bring forth this volume dedicated to Paul and his ideas.

Dan Kriegman

PREFACE
Judith Guss Teicholz, Ed.D.

It has been an honor for me to coordinate this book dedicated to the presentation of post-Freudian views on the repetition compulsion and its relationship to paradox, affect, and trauma.

It is with sadness that we realize that the late Paul Russell will not be able to reply to those who have discussed his two papers. There will be no one to correct their misunderstandings, and no one to argue with their differences. But I believe that his work has been read both lovingly and critically by each discussant, appreciated, agreed with and disagreed with on various points, clarified, amplified, and expanded. I can only hope that Paul Russell would be pleased with this recognition, if he were with us to experience it.

The book was sponsored by the Massachusetts Institute for Psychoanalysis (MIP), which was founded in 1987 as a center for the comparative study of psychoanalysis. Its faculty represents a broad cross-section of the different analytic paradigms.

The pleasure of being a primary editor of this project along with Daniel Kreigman was greatly enhanced by our dealings with all those who have contributed to its becoming a reality. Above all, we are very grateful to Deborah Russell for giving us permission to use two previously unpublished papers by Paul Russell. Paul was a founding member of MIP and provided active leadership as well as invaluable teaching and supervision of its candidates. His original voice and unique message are unclassifiable within any one analytic paradigm and push the bounds of any single theory.

Virginia Demos, George Fishman, Stephen Mitchell, and Arnold Modell have given freely of their scarce time, their prodigious creative talent, and their spirit of adventure to provide us with intellectually rigorous and vitally interesting discussions of Paul Russell's two papers. Additionally, Jane Leavy has generously constructed a theoretical/historical contextualization of his central ideas. Our appreciation of each of these analysts, for joining with us in this venture, is beyond words.

Our gratitude goes as well to Susan Fairfield who, in her role as associate editor, gave us the benefit of her literary and psychoanalytic backgrounds, her editing expertise, her standard of perfection, and her knowledge of the publishing world. She has put in time on this project that goes far beyond the call of duty and can only be interpreted as an act of love—for MIP, for psychoanalysis, and for this book.

127 Mt. Auburn Street
Cambridge, MA 02138

CONTRIBUTORS

PAUL L. RUSSELL, M.D., was Clinical Instructor in Psychiatry, Harvard Medical School; Associate Psychiatrist, Beth Israel Hospital; faculty member, Boston Psychoanalytic Institute; and faculty member and supervising analyst, Massachusetts Institute for Psychoanalysis.

JUDITH GUSS TEICHOLZ, Ed.D., is a faculty member and supervising analyst, Massachusetts Institute for Psychoanalysis and author of *The Postmodern Revolution in Psychoanalysis: Kohut, Loewald, and the New Relational Paradigms*, to be published by The Analytic Press in 1999.

DANIEL KRIEGMAN, Ph.D., is a faculty member, Massachusetts Institute for Psychoanalysis and co-author with Malcolm Slavin of *The Adaptive Design of the Human Psyche* (1992).

SUSAN FAIRFIELD is an editor and translator of psychoanalytic books.

E. VIRGINIA DEMOS, Ed.D., is Assistant Clinical Professor of Psychology, Harvard Medical School; a member of the medical staff of Austen Riggs Hospital, Stockbridge, MA; and faculty member, Massachusetts Institute for Psychoanalysis.

GEORGE G. FISHMAN, M.D., is Director of Psychotherapy Training at Beth Israel Deaconess Medical Center in Boston; Assistant Clinical Professor of Psychiatry, Harvard Medical School; training and supervising analyst, Boston Psychoanalytic

CONTRIBUTORS

Institute; and faculty member, Massachusetts Institute for Psychoanalysis.

JANE LEAVY, LICSW, is a clinical social worker and a graduate and faculty member of the Massachusetts Institute for Psychoanalysis. She is a consultant and supervisor at the Harvard University Mental Health Service and has a private practice in Newton, MA.

STEPHEN A. MITCHELL, Ph.D., is the editor of *Psychoanalytic Dialogues*; training and supervising analyst, William Alanson White Institute, New York; and faculty member and supervisor, New York University Postdoctoral Program. His latest book is *Influence and Autonomy in Psychoanalysis* (1997).

ARNOLD H. MODELL, M.D., is Clinical Professor of Psychiatry, Harvard Medical School, and training and supervising analyst, Boston Psychoanalytic Institute. His most recent books are *Other Times, Other Realities* (1990) and *The Private Self* (1994).

ONE

THE ROLE OF PARADOX IN THE REPETITION COMPULSION

Paul L. Russell, M.D.

Repetition is unavoidable. Life proceeds by repetitions, many times over, of the processes essential to it. The complex organization characteristic of life is repetitive: for example genetic encoding, cell division, patterns of growth and of learning. Habits are our collection, for better or worse, of repetitions. Repetition is inherent in any organized structure. We cannot live without repeating; in a sense, our repetitions are what we are.

The remarkable thing, however, is that life, and the growth characteristic of life, must necessarily be something other than repetition. In some peculiar way, the enterprise of life requires that one both remain the same and change, all at the same time. One is, and yet is not, who one was.

For some time now, we have had to assume that people come to understand their past not simply by remembering, describing, and reflecting upon it. Apparently, only through reliving the past can there come the kind of understanding that makes a difference. The reasons for this are complex and go to the heart of what is involved in human memory and human feeling. Freud (1914) framed the problem by saying that repeating, remembering, and working through are three stages of a continuous process. Our name for the earlier part of this difficult-to-understand but terribly important phenomenon is the repetition compulsion.

This is a most difficult, and fascinating, phenomenon that one can only assume lies at the very core of the problem of changing while remaining the same. As the name indicates, the repetition in this case is compulsive. It is a part of our experience that is familiar, utterly too familiar, but is repeated in ways that feel beyond our understanding and control. We find ourselves repeating that which, so far as we know, we would far rather not repeat.

For the most part, the repetition is of something actually, or potentially, painful. We do not complain, presumably, about pleasant repetitions. These we do our best to bring about and to enjoy. The repetition of something painful is another matter. We seem to be dealing here with some internal, systematic error that eludes our perception and control. In fact, the suspicion begins to dawn on us that the more painful the experience, the more we were injured by it, the more likely it is to be woven into something we find ourselves compulsively repeating. This is more than a little unsettling. It feels spooky; Freud used the word "daemonic." There is some powerful resistance that appears to operate against all efforts at learning to anticipate, to avoid, or to alter the painful repetition. The repetition compulsion is education-resistant.

We have a shorthand way of referring to this state of affairs. We say that the repetition compulsion and trauma are profoundly connected. Trauma can be thought of as anything that causes injury. And injury is anything that necessitates healing. Healing is a process of repair that as a general rule involves pain and dysfunction and requires mobilization of resources. The process, therefore, is costly. It consumes energy, and the organism is constrained to take time off from other enterprises. The idea, here, would be that the repetition compulsion functions as an attempt to heal. To whatever degree there is a systematic encroachment on the capacity to see things as they are, we can assume that this is because the present is being seen in terms of the past. It becomes a disorder in which memory is confused with perception. To whatever degree there has been trauma, it is inappropriately over-remembered and rendered as present experience. Trauma *is* that which gets compulsively repeated.

However, I would like to leave as an open question what exactly is the nature of the relationship between trauma and the repetition compulsion. One possibility would be that the original trauma takes a toll, creates an injury, and leaves a scar, the mark of which is its repetition. One would then want to investigate what exactly is the function of the repetition.

Another possibility would be that some kind of flaw, some particular sort of deficit in an individual, makes inevitable the repetition of a particular kind of painful situation. In this case, the repetition compulsion might be said to exist before the trauma takes place. George Fishman (personal communication) has said that the repetition is not necessarily a repetition of anything that ever actually happened.

It may indeed be that the association between trauma and the repetition compulsion does not explain anything at all. This might be simply an organizing assumption we make, totally without evidence: a daemonic myth. I do submit, however, that the repetition compulsion is a fact. It is, I think, universal. It is not always easy to see, especially in oneself. The temptation is overwhelming to blame something, anything, outside ourselves.

In the long run, it is only the fact of the repetition itself that has any hope of making us realize that the odds of it happening by chance, or indeed from any factor at all outside ourselves, reach the vanishing point.

Psychotherapists have a unique opportunity for observation, since transference is a species of the repetition compulsion. One can think of psychopathology in general as the operation of the repetition compulsion. We can only assume that it is a much deeper and larger part of who we are than we have any way of seeing. I would like, however, to insert an asterisk here. I think that we need to notice the nature of the relationship we have with those persons around whom, with whom, and through whom we repeat.

Why do people repeat? One possibility is that we do so in an attempt at belated active mastery: bad as it is, it's better if I do it than if it's done to me. This may have to do with the idea of trauma as an overload that has to be worked off in some kind of piecemeal, repeated way. Perhaps it has to do with the attachment to the familiar and to the devils one knows. Perhaps there is a hidden wish, a covert perverse pleasure, in the repetition. Perhaps it is an archaic attempt at control, or a quest for a needed but lost relationship. Another possibility involves the architecture of memory. George Santayana's (1954) observation that "those who cannot remember the past are condemned to relive it" (p. 82) would seem to suggest this. The repetition compulsion goes to the heart of the capacity to remember and the capacity to feel.

Let me suggest that it has a great deal to do with how we feel. Or, more exactly, what we cannot feel. The idea would be that the repetition occurs in lieu of something we cannot yet feel, a kind of affective incompetence. Given the failure to feel, the rest—the "compulsive" repetitions—happen necessarily, mathematically, if you will. As one of my patients said, "You have to keep doing it until you get it right!"

This matter of the internal mathematics of affective competency might be illustrated by the learning of a sport, for example skiing. This is a very vivid metaphor for me. I learned to ski late enough in life for it to be an actively remembered trauma. The competence in this case is a cerebellar one. The general theorem is that the ratio of competence to incompetence defines a topography that is specific to the individual attempting the task.

The only thing that keeps a pair of skis from being a totally frictionless surface hurtling headlong down the hill is the fact that they have edges. Easier, but relatively inefficient, is the use of the inside edge of each ski, the snowplow. More difficult, but ultimately offering more control, is the use in parallel of the complementary edges, the left for a left turn, the right for a right. Now the mathematics are that if you do not edge, you will fall. There are only three basic choices: edge, fall, or stay off the hill. The hill *coerces* either competence, or a repetition—falling. When one is in the middle of the repetition, it feels perverse, malignant, and evil. It is hard, at the moment, to apprehend what one is doing wrong.

One particularly bad day, I found myself attacked repeatedly by the Snow Snake, the same one that grabs people by the ankle and makes them fall. Put yourself now in the position of my ski instructor. He has been sketching out the borders of my competence. The fall occurs just here, at the moment when the hill, plus the speed, plus the turn demand just such a certain movement, which I cannot yet do. And my incapacity to do just that movement defines, quite exactly, a particular topography of steepness of hill, speed, and sharpness of curve that will necessarily spell *fall*. After some practice runs, I begin to get the hang of that particular movement. But we then move to a steeper hill. And a new final common incompetence is defined. I meet the Snow Snake once again.

I will be told, for example, that I am leaning too much into the hill. "The edges you must use," the instructor will say, "are the uphill edges. If you catch a downhill edge, you fall. Now to do that, your upper body has to lean not into the hill, but away from it, into the valley, into space." This, I discover, is terrifying, unnatural, and against every instinct.

The cerebellum functions, for the most part, unconsciously. The need for a new competence coerces a raising into consciousness of successive feeling–thinking–doing sequences that will, slowly, broaden the topography, that is, establish a new ratio of competence versus repetition. Notice that with competence occurs a transformation of affect: terror into exhilaration. A skilled ski instructor will figure out the next most critical as-yet-unmastered task and can suggest ways, not apparent to the learner, in which there can be bridges to this from what is already known. Notice also that each steeper hill, each sharper, faster turn, will necessitate a temporary return of the old terrified, unnatural feeling. One must discover anew, at each fresh juncture, that there are other ways than those that one has been used to.

Now I'd like you to notice one last thing. Let us suppose that instead of the expectable, gradual development of the ability to ski, there occurs instead a residual pocket of incompetence that seems to resist all efforts. Other congruent areas of growing skill will demarcate this one island into high relief. "You persist in favoring that ankle," the ski instructor might say. "Was it ever injured?" Or even, "There's nothing about what we're doing that ought to bother you. Are you afraid of something?"

To start off with, it cannot be known what causes the persistent repetition of failure, only that it occurs in an increasingly sharply demarcated area of dysfunction that itself suggests, more and more pointedly, some kind of earlier injury around that area. Again, it is quite arbitrary at which point something ceases to be simply a lingering pocket of difficulty and becomes instead a systematic dysfunction pointing to trauma. Sooner or later, however, if the individual wants to ski, or live life, the hill forces the issue. One assumes the existence of injury because the hallmarks are there; that is to say, the sensitized area evokes pain, dysfunction, and a sapping of energy, all over and above what the situation itself would seem to account for. One assumes the existence of injury because addressing one's attention and resources to the healing process is the only thing at that point that will work.

I am now going to try to build the case specifically as it relates to the capacity to feel. To do this, I want to say some things about feelings and what they are, or at least some of the necessary life functions they perform. But first I want to go back to the asterisk I inserted earlier, namely the *relationship* between the individual repeating, on the one hand, and the significant others with whom he or she goes through the repetition, on the other. My view is that this is an intensely paradoxical relationship.

The repetition compulsion would seem to be two things. One is the nucleus of an organized system of affective incompetence, a dysfunctional feeling system. It is also an attempt to continue an interrupted relationship in the service of the emotional growth that was earlier broken off. It is the scar tissue of the injury to the capacity to feel. There are at least four paradoxes that seem to surround and invest every act of repetition. These seem to be essential paradoxes in the growth of human feeling, because they so closely describe and demarcate the repetition compulsion: Is this me or is this you? Did I do this, or was it done to me? Is this now, or was it then? Can I choose what I feel?

The treatment process is necessarily risky. Some treatments clearly carry a risk of psychosis or suicide. The probability is that every treatment carries a potential for psychosis or suicide at some point. But this is not the only risk. We can make the point much more generally. The risk of psychotherapy has to do with the nature of the repetition compulsion. We cannot learn to stop repeating in advance of the repetition. The repetition compulsion has already resisted every attempt at learning from experience. It is by definition those parts of our behavior, of ourselves, that we would most want to change, but cannot. What happens, at every opportunity to change, is a repeat. In order to *choose* not to repeat, one has to have been aware of and lived through those parts of one's experience where the risk of repetition is greatest. The risk, therefore, is that this will happen in the treatment as well, but at a time and a place and in a way in which the stakes are much higher than they are otherwise, precisely because of the attachment, in reality, to the therapist.

It is as if things cannot be real, and the patient will not feel psychotherapy means anything, until the treatment situation becomes so much like a dangerous part of the patient's past that there is in fact a real risk of a repeat of the past. I had this in mind when I said before that it is especially in the nature of trauma that it repeat. Freud's succinct but profound idea was that every finding is in fact a refinding.

The transference, remember, is not something the patient is play-acting. There are at least two elements of the transference that carry genuine risk. One is that the patient cannot feel any real alternative. Things we cannot feel are not likely to happen; things are repeated because that's the way it feels. The other is that the patient focuses on those aspects of us that in fact do recapture the past, real parts of ourselves that do, to some degree, prove their point. However odious, this aspect needs to be located in us, and for us to try to disown or disavow it, to ascribe it all to "transference," is to sever the patient's emotional connection with us. The only thing that works is negotiation, namely a negotiation around whether things have to happen the same way this time (cf. Loewald 1971).

This particular negotiation is one of the most difficult that life offers. The compulsion to repeat occurs with an urgency that appears to surpass all others. And yet there is also within every repetition the wish to be stopped. There is the wish that the therapist (or somebody) protect the patient from the ravages of the repetition compulsion. We see this as a kind of rage preceding and defending against a grief reaction. The grief is real: it is grief over the loss of life possibilities. This negotiation represents the most difficult part of the treatment process. The patient finds in us precisely those aspects of his or her past that make the repeat of trauma a real possibility and risk the interruption, or the end, of the treatment process. Usually the two go together—the trauma is the loss of connectedness. To say why this is so, I would like to recap something of what I said several years ago about urgencies and crises of attachment (Russell 1981).

One of the major reasons negotiation is so integral to the development of affective competence is that affect and intention are profoundly connected. Every feeling contains a wish. Clearly one of the things that impressed Freud about sexuality was that an entire physiological system of arousal was involved, with complex interplays of excitement versus inhibition and repression. Inhibition represented the more competent, conscious mechanism of control. Another effective, but far more costly, mechanism of control was repression. The cost was neurosis. Sexuality was so elegant a paradigm of the development of the capacity to wish, that it is understandable how long it was thought to be the primary wish or basic drive. Freud added one other wish to the roster of basic drives before he died: aggression. The conflict model he developed around drive and defense for sexuality served quite well for aggression also, although even today we are somewhat less certain about the psychoaggressive stages of development than we are about the original psychosexual model.

Freud saw the mind—more specifically, the ego—as the container of urgencies. There is, then, a necessary and continuous tension between the press for action, on the one hand, and the need for delay in the service of competence, on the other. I think today we can say that a relationship is more primary, both in a chronological and a conceptual sense, as the container of human urgencies. However, it is as true today as when Freud first formulated the theory, that conflict is inherent in choice. What is more clear today is the complexity of the paradoxical relationship between the interpersonal negotiations and the intrapsychic ones.

Heinz Kohut (1977) shares the view that some wishes are more basic, more primary than others, although for him the basic drive is not sex or aggression but the need for a cohesive sense of self, from which sex and aggression are themselves derivative. I would like to suggest that every wish contains its own species of drive, its own conflictual epigenetic history. Every feeling carries with it some quotient of urgency, a probability greater than before that that particular something will happen. Any feeling serves the function of a potential preparation for an act.

Affect, the capacity to feel, performs other basic functions as well. In addition to intention, every affect performs a cognitive function. In the older literature, the word *affect* carries a clear connotation of accompanying bodily changes, that is to say, autonomic ones. This bias was so profound that before the time of Papez and MacLean the two things were thought to be neuroanatomically very separate; the emotions were thought to be autonomic phenomena, distal to the cerebrospinal system, and cognition an event that took place in the cerebral cortex. Later research and reflection draw the two much closer together, both conceptually and neuroanatomically. Functionally, they cannot be separated.

Freud (1926) saw anxiety as performing a unique signal function to the ego. Bibring (1954) extended this by suggesting that depression also served as signal to the ego, and Zetzel (1970) saw the capacity to experience both anxiety and depression as a critical measure of ego strength. Melanie Klein (1952) had earlier suggested a kind of epigenetic unfolding of affective competence, in which the capacity to experience depression was what allowed one to relinquish the reality-distorting mechanisms of denial and projection. The crucial concept here is that all affects serve as signals, as indicators of reality.

Affects also serve a communicative function; they are signals not only to us, but also from us to other people. Every affect communicates its particular disposition. Affects thus perform a basic attachment function. The result of all of the above is some shaping, some alteration of the nature and structure of attachment. As Arnold Modell (1984) puts it, "Affects are object-seeking" (p. 21). And, finally, all affects perform a crucial developmental function. This is implicit in the concept of the repetition compulsion. The essential negotiation with each repetition is whether it is an exact repetition, costly to the degree to which it relives the past in lieu of the present, or whether something new occurs in the direction of more successful wishing, clearer signal function, and deeper attachment—in short, the wherewithal for greater competency.

Now, it would appear that the experience of paradox is one of the vital signs of emotional development. Another way of saying this is that the capacity to tolerate paradox is a measure of ego strength (see Kumin 1987). Insofar as we understand anything, we attempt to make our understanding consistent (that is, without contradiction) and complete (because what we leave out might be the most important thing). But paradox shatters the attempt to be both consistent and complete. We cannot live with it. Yet there are times when what we seek, what we require, can be found only by ceasing to struggle and letting the paradox teach us.

Let me give you an example of a genuine logical paradox: the barber shaves all and only those who do not shave themselves. Who shaves the barber? There are only two possibilities. Either he shaves himself or he doesn't. But, according to the terms of the definition, if he does, then he doesn't; and if he doesn't, then he does. Another example: a card has written on it: "The statement on the other side of this card is false." You turn it over, and it reads: "The statement on the other side of this card is true." Most of us are able to live our lives without having to take things like this seriously anyplace outside of a book of puzzles or some occasional after-dinner games. The barber paradox, however, or one very like it, is famous. I'll tell you as much as I can about that, in a moment.

The Role of Paradox

The historian and philosopher of science, Thomas Kuhn, has written a book called *The Structure of Scientific Revolutions* (1970), in which he offers a helpful perspective on our problem. Science, he believes, does not somehow get closer and closer to truth by accumulating more and more facts and theories, as if truth were some kind of asymptote, some kind of ideal that we gradually approach. Insofar as any enterprise becomes truly scientific, it does so through revolutions. A genuinely new advance cannot simply be added to existing knowledge; there is necessarily a clash, a crisis of theory that at least in some measure destroys the old, like an insect having to crack and shed the old exoskeleton in order to grow the new.

For example, the Copernican solar-system world view had a revolutionary impact upon the earth-centered Ptolemaic system. We might call the old Ptolemaic system more self-centered, more narcissistic, but Kuhn's point is that periods of orthodoxy followed by revolution constitute the natural and necessary evolution of science and not some kind of psychological or sociological overlay. Or, put another way, the psychological and sociological is a necessary and integral part of the evolution of science. The very cohesion, elegance, simplicity, and inclusiveness that a theory works so hard to achieve are what in the end make it vulnerable, make it unable to accommodate anomaly.

The revolution begins with the noticing of anomaly. The old way of looking at things does not account for *something* that up until this point has been ignored, tolerated, distorted, or accounted for in a way that turns out to be contradictory. It is taking the anomaly seriously that, in Kuhn's view, leads to a paradigm, a new way of measuring, assessing, discovering, and ordering phenomena. At this point one is forced either to reject the existence of the anomaly and the paradigm that attempts to explain it, or else to discard the entire older conceptual apparatus that made the anomaly anomalous. We see here a familiar oscillating tension between consistency and completeness. To understand anything, we have no choice but to capture as much of both consistency and completeness as we possibly can. But somehow the one is always at the expense of the other, and eventually, as the two come together, any theoretical system seems to deliver the anomaly that will eventually overthrow it.

I mentioned the barber paradox a moment ago. What I think is fascinating is that this internal dialectic between consistency and completeness occurs not just in laboratories, in the outer world of scientific observation. It occurs even—and especially—in pure subjects like mathematics and logic, in the mind of the thinker before leaving the armchair. A priori, analytic systems such as these are immune from correction by any external empirical anomalous observations. In this case, the nemesis is paradox.

Paradox became a very real and very insoluble problem to Russell and Whitehead in *Principia Mathematica* (1938). Had they managed to resolve it, they might have achieved what surely would have been the most elegant piece of intellectual synthesis since Newton. The story is a fascinating one. Russell and Whitehead attempted to reduce all of mathematics, and thereby all that was supported by mathematics, to the language of logic. The concepts of class and description were to replace concepts of number and the various mathematical operations. In order to be complete they had to allow for any conceivable class, any conceivable description. What, then, about a hypothetical class such as the class of all classes that do not include themselves as a member? Does it belong to itself, or not? It's the barber paradox, except that in this case it makes a real difference, and there is no way out. At this point there was no choice except either to make some kind of ad hoc, arbitrary rule against paradoxical classes, or else to await the arrival of a synthesizing system that could somehow underlie, explain, or go beyond the paradox. That's where matters stood until Kurt Gödel proved that there could be no such system (see Nagel and Newman 1958). For any system, it is impossible to be both logically consistent and complete—that is, without paradox. A simple contradiction is something that can be discovered, sooner or later, to be either true or not true, without expense to the rest of the system. A paradox is *something that the coherence and consistency of the entire rest of the system require to be both true and not true, a contradiction from which there is no escape without the destruction of the system.*

I am not a mathematician, logician, or philosopher. However, I was struck by the similarity to what happens in a crisis of the treatment process, and I wondered whether it might be possible to frame—what shall we call them?—the paradoxes of emotional development. What I take, rightly or wrongly, from Kuhn, Russell and Whitehead, and Gödel, is that for any conceptual grid, for any framework of understanding, to the extent that one comes close to coherence, consistency, and completeness, one can expect to encounter, one necessarily delivers, a paradox that is specific to that level of understanding. Whatever the inadequacies of the conceptual grid, this paradox fills the spectrum of awareness in a way that makes more or less revolutionary overthrow the only way of expanding to allow the perception of new phenomena. The only entry that can be made into the relatively airtight older system is through paradox. This is the individual's only way of knowing that he can't have it both ways. It could be thought of, teleologically, as a stimulus, a goad to the mind to expand the containing framework of understanding that goes on as long as there is life, feeling, and thinking.

One has the feeling, as one struggles with the compulsion to repeat both personally and professionally, of experiencing at close hand the basic paradox of life, namely the need to change and to remain the same, both at the same time. Real change, both for our patients and for us, arises from within a repetition. Patients are terrified of the power they have to create a repetition and to evoke repetitions of our own that make us—however limited the context and in however limited a fashion—in fact wish to detach from them.

In our work, the unfolding of the repetition necessarily represents an acute crisis of relatedness. The problem is intensely paradoxical: to the extent that affective connectedness has in fact made the relationship a usably safe one, the patient has recreated the risk of a loss of that connectedness, precisely because it has been safe to do so. The therapist's empathic connectedness simply underlines the problem. It is precisely this that the patient feels the need to defend against. I think that this problem is best described as negotiating the continuation of the relationship. The reason it cannot be interpreted is that what we are negotiating is something that has never happened before, namely the experience of loss and detachment in the presence of attachment, of containment.

The continuation of the relationship at this point depends upon the therapist. It won't happen if the therapist is simply waiting for the patient to "work through the transference." The reason is that the patient needs the therapist to be equally in touch with very dissonant pieces of reality that have not yet come together. These include awareness of the patient's past; awareness of what it is the patient is struggling not to feel, think, or say about the therapist; and awareness, also, of how it is that the therapist does in fact play this, until now, unspoken role because of the therapist's own needs and repetitions.

There is no real treatment process that does not include some piece of therapy for the therapist. This is not by design or intent; it is simply a part of any growth relationship. I have said before that the major resistance to the treatment process is the therapist's resistance. The therapist's resistance to change, to modifying or negotiating an alternative to her own repetition for the sake of continuing the treatment process, is the first major piece of that resistance. And there is one other piece of reality that the therapist must be aware of, even if it is hard to feel; this is the patient's need for the treatment relationship to continue, for the therapist to continue to be the therapist.

The patient often harbors the fantasy, which the therapist sometimes shares, that if the therapist can avoid the repetition, some kind of corrective emotional experience can occur. The thing that is in fact traumatizing is not the repetition, which has to happen in some measure, but the therapist's not being in touch with what he or she feels. The failure to feel on the part of the therapist does in fact recreate a context-specific loss of connectedness.

We are talking here about what is often called countertransference. There are two difficulties with this term: one is that it suggests that the therapist's transference is somehow only in response to, or counter to, the patient's. The therapist's countertransference in fact comes just as much from the therapist's past life, from the therapist's own compulsion to repeat, as it does from the patient. The second is that some of the earlier writing suggests that countertransference has to be analyzed or somehow controlled lest it interfere with the treatment process. The problem is that there's no way it won't interfere; it is inevitably woven into the treatment crisis.

I prefer to call it the therapist's urgency. Urgency is part of life. We do, in fact, try to keep our needs for our patients to a minimum, but in the long run patients need our urgencies just as much as they need our empathy. This is the only way we have of understanding the crisis, of beginning to feel where and how the loss of relatedness occurs. This turns out to be the second major piece of resistance on the part of the therapist. We resist feeling ourselves what things were really like for the patient. We tell ourselves we know their history, but it is not possible to do this work without resistance against feeling the pain. And it's no mystery that what we do not want to feel with our patients bears directly on what we resist in ourselves. What we have to ask of ourselves is nothing other than what we hope the treatment process may make possible for the patient, namely that the urgencies be used, not in the service of repeating, but as a way of feeling what could not be felt before.

Therapists have their own past and their own repetitions. There is no way that this is not part of the negotiation. It would be much easier if the patient were the only one who repeated in the service of remembering and working through, and the therapist simply understood by drawing on memories within him- or herself of things already worked through. There are just enough not-so-difficult treatments where things are more or less like this that we hold them as a model, albeit a limited one, to ourselves, and try not to deviate from this model. However, the difficult treatment forces us to widen our experience, to recognize that there are parts of ourselves, much more than the troublesome parts of our patients, that we do not yet understand. Some experiences are so scorching, some feelings so frightening or painful, that, at whatever cost, the patient will know far more about them than we do. They do not need us to know immediately. But they do need us to know that we do not know. The most important source of resistance in the treatment process is the therapist's resistance to what the patient feels.

The capacity to feel never develops in isolation. It is a negotiation, a crucial, life-sustaining negotiation that emerges from within a relationship. Rorey Anscombe (1981) has said the organ of mind necessarily includes another person. It is this crucial affective negotiation that makes possible the treatment process. The therapeutic leverage derives from two sources, which must come together. The first is the perception on the part of the patient, made vivid by the unfolding of the transference, of his own contribution to the way the world feels. This occurs in a situation where it is in fact safe to transfer. The second comes from the fact that the therapist is, in reality, different from the original object from whom the transference derives. This is not so much disclosed as simply perceived and felt. These two are interlocking events. The very fact of the safety is, paradoxically, what allows the repetition to unfold with the degree of risk that it necessarily entails. The therapeutic leverage comes from the therapist's allowing the patient, in a non-urgent way, to experience both at the same time. The therapist must negotiate to be both the person(s) with whom the initial negotiation failed and the person with whom it might possibly be different. This amounts to negotiating the possibility of containment in the treatment situation. This is, by virtually any reckoning, impossible. For it to happen at all depends upon the growth in both therapist and patient of the capacity to feel. All of this amounts to both parties feeling in full measure why, for each, and each for his own reasons, the relationship cannot possibly safely survive, and yet it does so because all of this is felt, and the relationship survives.

I referred earlier to two possibilities: one that the repetition was of actual trauma, and the other that the problem lies totally within the individual. Both are true. Or, put another way, the paradox of the repetition compulsion is that one must negotiate one's attachments assuming that one is totally responsible for everything that happens, at the same time that one creates the possibility for someone else to make a difference.

The repetition compulsion is an invitation to a crisis. The repetition can occur alone, but the crisis cannot. If there is no significant independent connection with an important other person, the repetition is stereotyped, highly predictable, virtually automatic, and safe. If there is a significant emotional connection to someone in the present real world, for example a therapist, a crisis occurs that amounts to the person being forced to change the way she feels in order to be in a relationship. This process, however, carries real risk. We refer to it as the regression of the treatment process. This amounts to making the situation enough like the past to virtually insure a repetition of an emotionally crippling loss, and yet holding out the possibility, at least, of a negotiation for feeling an attachment in the service of growth.

There is, I think, such a thing as a logic of feelings. The trouble is, there is no calculus and no computer that will help, because understanding the logic requires the capacity to feel. Paradoxically, the only thing that can help is the very problem we have been struggling with: the repetition compulsion.

At this point, I would like to remind you of the ways in which paradox acts as a spur, a goad, a stimulus to the mind to expand the framework of understanding. Let me repeat it, but thinking this time not so much of logical systems as of the capacity to feel. This is a never-ending process. Whatever we can organize as coherent and complete is to that degree predictable, controllable, and comfortable. But the very attempt to cast our awareness in terms that are both coherent and complete delivers a paradox that marks the limits of our understanding and fractures the structure at the point of its greatest weakness. This is as true in the realm of the capacity to feel as it is anywhere else. In fact there is no essential difference; it is all of a piece. Feelings *are* our spectrum of awareness. The repetition compulsion serves as a reminder that we have not yet found a way to feel differently.

REFERENCES

Anscombe, R. (1981). Philosophical critique of Schafer's action language. *International Journal of Psycho-Analysis* 62:225–247.

Bibring, E. (1954). Psychoanalysis and the dynamic psychotherapies. *Journal of the American Psychoanalytic Association* 2:745–763.

——— (1953). The mechanism of depression. In *Affective Disorders*, ed. P. Greenacre, pp. 13–48. New York: International Universities Press.

Freud, S. (1914). Remembering, repeating, and working-through. *Standard Edition* 12:145–156.

——— (1926). Inhibitions, symptoms, and anxiety. *Standard Edition* 20:77–172.

Klein, M. (1952). Some theoretical conclusions regarding the emotional life of the infant. In *Developments in Psycho-Analysis*, ed. M. Klein, P. Heimann, S. Isaacs, and J. Riviere, pp. 195–236. London: Hogarth.

Kohut, H. (1977). *The Restoration of the Self.* Madison, CT: International Universities Press.

Kuhn, T. S. (1970). *The Structure of Scientific Revolutions*, 2nd ed. Chicago: University of Chicago Press.

Kumin, I. M. (1987). Developmental aspects of opposites and paradox. *International Review of Psycho-Analysis* 5:477–484.

Loewald, H. (1971). Some considerations on repetition and repetition compulsion. *International Journal of Psycho-Analysis* 52:59–66.

Modell, A. H. (1984). *Psychoanalysis in a New Context.* New York: International Universities Press.

Nagel, E., and Newman, J. R. (1958). *Gödel's Proof.* New York: New York University Press.

Russell, B., and Whitehead, A. N. (1938). *Principia Mathematica.* New York: Norton.

Russell, P. L. (1981). Emotional growth and crises of attachment. Unpublished manuscript.

Santayana, G. (1954). *The Life of Reason.* New York: Scribner.

Zetzel, E. (1970). *The Capacity for Emotional Growth.* London: Hogarth.

TWO

TRAUMA AND THE COGNITIVE FUNCTION OF AFFECTS

Paul L. Russell, M.D.

> At some point you are going to have to decide that the most important things you have are your feelings.
> —DON FERN

*T*rauma and the repetition compulsion appear to be specific to one another. Why is this?

One of the most intriguing things to notice in the development of anyone engaged in the enterprise of treatment, whether as patient, therapist, or teacher, is the way one returns, again and again, to the idea of the repetition compulsion. One can make a case for its being the most important conceptual tool Freud gave us, underlying all of the others. What seems to recur is the question: Why do people repeat over and over again the same situation, the same feelings, the same trauma, no matter how painful, how maladaptive, how injurious?

Whatever has been overwhelming, assaultive, rendering the individual helpless to respond, is somehow necessarily repeated. Perhaps this occurs because of a need for belated active mastery, a need to work off the trauma somehow, or perhaps the trauma touches off some kind of basic masochism, a death wish, that makes the individual repeat.

Whatever the reason, I think there is little doubt about the phenomenon and its absolute centrality. Let me, to begin with, make the general working assumption that the repetition compulsion and psychopathology amount to the same thing. To whatever degree there is a systematic encroachment on the capacity to see things as they are, we can assume that this is because the present is being seen in terms of the past. We might call it a disorder of memory. To whatever degree there has been trauma, it is inappropriately over-remembered. I would like to suggest that this disorder of memory is affectively determined. It amounts to an injury to the capacity to feel.

In my paper "The Theory of the Crunch" (1975), I wanted to understand the way in which the crises in the treatment of the more difficult patient were repetitions. They were repetitions of the injuries to, and failures of, the capacity to relate and were then delivered into the treatment situation as a crisis of, and a threat to, the treatment relationship itself. The stress that this places on the containing function of treatment suggested that the original injury occurred in the absence of a similar containing function in the past.

In my paper "Beyond the Wish" (1976), I wanted to see in what ways this mechanism is a general one; that is, can psychopathology in general be understood as failure of containment—of a wish? One initial problem of the language of wishing is the departure from more familiar terminology, such as id versus ego, instinctual drive versus defense. A wish then becomes utterly general: whatever can give meaning to, can define, an act. The advantage I hoped for was to leave the particular nature and function of the wish entirely open to discovery, something demonstrable by the treatment process itself. In other words, if the entire matter of instinctual vicissitudes, repression, symptom formation, and psychopathology can apply to *any* wish, not just the sexual one, the focus shifts in an important way. What Freud then provides is not simply a theory of the vicissitudes of certain kinds of wishes, for examples sexual or aggressive; it is more importantly a statement about the ways in which the capacity to render a wish can itself be subject to injury.

This shift in focus seems to me to point up two things: first, the importance of the containing function in the development of the capacity to wish, and therefore the importance of reality. In other words, wishes that fail to be rendered are stunted because *in reality*, at some point in time, the existence of the wish significantly threatened the conditions of life. The sexual and aggressive wishes are paradigms. The containing of these wishes becomes, in reality, the shared imperative task of an entire family, not just the child. Containing the wish means postponement of consummation when the consequences would, in reality, be too costly, but in a way that allows for full use of the developing wish later on in the service of life. Failure of containment is traumatizing. It is traumatizing because the individual must attempt to do the containing himself, but in a way that costs him the capacity, later on, to render the wish. Real containment occurs, to begin with, only in a relationship, and the capacity to render the wish later on depends upon the taking in of the earlier, actual competency in the relationship. The essence of trauma is that, without containment, the wish costs the individual the relationship.

And thus we come full circle: trauma and the repetition compulsion are specific to one another. I would like to explore the ways in which this unfolds: the ways in which the capacity to wish, the capacity to feel, the capacity to think, and the capacity to act all converge and are all injured, and in a manner that necessarily repeats the trauma.

One of the difficulties in understanding childhood traumata, when treating the adult, is the fact that a great deal has intervened in the meantime. There is a lot to learn, therefore, when the trauma is recent. Sarah Haley (1974) has spoken about her work in the treatment of traumatized Vietnam War veterans who have committed atrocities. Her experience is such that she can tell, some time in advance, when a patient is going to begin to bring himself to describe an atrocity. There is a dread and foreboding, and a steeling oneself against it, along with the sense that it is absolutely imperative to hear what is going to be described. Then, as the horror of the act emerges, the therapist is thrown back: "This cannot be! He is a monster! No human could have done this!" But the treatment process requires that the therapist be able to feel, "I could well have done that." It does not have to be said, just felt, but there is a clear difference between being able and not able to feel it. And the patient can tell. No matter how experienced he may be, it is always in some measure costly to the therapist each time the horror is felt. Yet the treatment process requires that this be done. One cannot understand the trauma unless one can feel what the patient felt.

Now, there are two aspects, of the many rich things Haley presented, that I would like you to think about, because the question would be whether they represent essential aspects of every trauma. The first is that the trauma appears to reside at an interface, both sides of which are necessary components of the injury. One side is a reality situation that is assaultive, overwhelming. The other side is a wish that has destructive potential and becomes, in some measure, actualized. The trauma, insofar as it continues to live as a psychic injury and to sap the individual's energies by repeating itself, weaves together both components. The trauma for the veteran includes both the reality of the Vietnam War and all that it did to him, as well as the reality of the destructive potential of the veteran's own actualized wish to kill.

The second factor I would like you to think about is the loneliness. Haley described poignantly the loneliness of the veteran returning home from having participated in an unpopular war, utterly without sanction. And yet this loneliness is only a tangible screen for a more scorching internal loneliness. The person feels alone, destitute, without resources or sanction, and disintegrated to the extent that there is a convergence of two realities, inner and outer, the wish and the event. The result is that the traumatizing texture of this interface is repeated, in some measure alone, apart, even from the rest of himself.

The capacity of the therapist to feel both realities appears to make a critical difference to this traumatizing texture. At this point, I would like simply to note the phenomenon, call it containment, and pose the question: How does it occur?

Kai Erikson (1976) has given us a poignant and beautiful description of the Buffalo Creek disaster. Let me remind you of some of the elements of the trauma, of the "psychic concussion" that he noted. There was a sense of being overwhelmed, assaulted, as if being attacked by a savage animal. The person will say, quite literally and exactly, "I cannot stand it" and then feel numb, sapped, drained, as if a part of the vital substance had been torn away. There is a sense of disorientation in time, place, and person. The clock stops at the time of the disaster, and in some important sense life ceases. The place where one is becomes strange, unconnected, without direction, without attachment, lost and homeless, even though at home. And, finally, the persons are not themselves. Divorce rates go up, things are not the same as they used to be, and there is a sense of suspicion, paranoia, and loneliness.

Erikson's suggestion was that we not think of the trauma simply in terms of the individual physical and psychic assault, terrible though that was. He noted that an essential dimension of the trauma consisted of the rupture, the rent to the cohesive social fabric, the sense of connectedness that made the Buffalo Creek community an organic whole. There was a loss of the containing envelope of the illusion of safety provided by human attachments, and it was the assault to this, to the containing structure, that constituted the trauma.

Here again, let me simply note the phenomenon of containment—in this case the containment of a human community—and ask: What is this, and how does it happen?

The work done by Sharon McCombie and her colleagues in the Rape Crisis Program* sheds some valuable light on the problem of the interface of inner and outer reality. Rape is the paradigm of violent assault, in which the victim is passive and helpless. There is no question of wish on the part of the victim. And yet an important part of the trauma is the guilt. The victim is herself compelled to raise this question. In other words, the trauma not only distorts and colors the future; the past is also retroactively charged and invested with new significance. Events, feelings, fantasies, and wishes of the past become retroactively informed by the trauma. The guilt, which appears to be general, can be thought of as a retroactive magical attempt at con-

---

Editor's Note: Dr. Russell's literary executors regret that they are unable to supply the title and date of this presentation.

trol ("If I had not been so seductive, it would not have happened"). Even if there are elements of the seductive wish, the essence of the trauma is the violent rupture of the envelope of safety, in which the person in retrospect thinks of the wish and the event as controlling one another. The trauma takes a toll on the individual's capacity to feel and distinguish inner and outer reality. It is as if the only way to make sense of an otherwise meaningless, horrifying assault is to cast it in terms of shame and guilt. The trauma forces an emotional regression to earlier issues and earlier ways of dealing with them.

I would like to mention one other property of trauma that is suggested by these examples. And that is that a significant trauma can be an organizing focus, a kind of prototype, that serves as a filter, a screen, an interpretation of earlier situations and events. It informs retroactively. Kai Erikson suggested this in comparing the Buffalo Creek disaster with the chronic trauma of poverty.

The examples we have been discussing up to now are ones that highlight the factor of trauma. They are, in other words, at one end of the complemental series (which will be discussed later). Also important would be the other end of that series, namely what the individual herself brings to the situation. It is this other end of the series that makes the discussion of early trauma so difficult. For example, there are times when someone's further growth and development require a trauma.

Let us now see whether some of these characteristics of recent trauma apply also to earlier trauma and to the repetition compulsion in general. Suppose you have been working with someone over a reasonable period of time. You and the patient know enough about each other to have done some useful work. This means that there is at least one major context in which you and the patient experience enough trust with each other to feel that the treatment relationship holds the promise of growth. But inevitably woven into that growth will be something like the following: a series of dreams, or some memories, or some triggering events, or perhaps nothing in particular one can point to, will herald an emerging feeling that, as it unfolds, carries with it the charge of an invitation to injury. The relationship becomes clouded, dense, murky, and somehow interpreted in a different way. It becomes increasingly difficult for things to remain as they had been until now. The patient feels that before anything else can happen, it has to be decided, right now, whether you, the therapist, are or are not somehow participating in, or creating, a fresh version of a familiar injury.

It is not at all certain that the old trust and good feeling will carry the day. In fact, the patient seems specifically to require something additional, something tangible, from the therapist to help decide the issue, and the therapist is placed in an awkward dilemma. To provide the something additional feels crazy; on some level it fulfills a function that should not be necessary and would not be were it not for the patient's psychopathology. And yet not to do something runs the risk of injury to the treatment relationship.

The therapist oscillates between wondering whether the patient has a paranoid streak and remembering that there are a great many internal and external factors from the patient's past that converge to make it, at first barely conceivable, then understandable, and finally inevitable, that it should feel just now the way it does. The therapist feels under the gun. To the extent that the patient is (however momentarily) paranoid, the only response that seems to work is total, complete, unchallenging empathy. And yet the therapist also feels that all an empathic response will do, ultimately, is postpone some necessary, painful, hard work.

Perhaps what is needed is empathy *plus* some critical difference in feeling and perception that the therapist suggests. But this goes beyond total, complete empathy and will be felt, to some degree, as an attack, as an injury, as distancing, as a loss of the relationship.

We have here a clash of two different realities, each with its own logic. Entering into the one totally precludes participating in the other. Rorey Anscombe (1981) has written a paper that elegantly and beautifully describes the ways in which the differences in logic, in modality, have a mutually impenetrable quality. Paranoia is an example, but every transference is paranoid. Insofar as the trauma is repeated, it is contained by the paranoia that is specific to it.

It is hard to know how to talk about what is going on, but one thing is certain, and that is that there is a very real crisis in the treatment relationship. One of three things has to happen: 1) There is some kind of compromise that amounts to protecting the relationship from the disruptive dissonance of the two realities. This usually means symptom formation. 2) The relationship in some way suffers; it is attenuated or broken off. 3) The relationship somehow contains the two realities in a way that, apparently, failed to occur at some earlier point in time, with traumatizing effect. In other words, there is a healing of the injury.

It appears that in talking about containment in this way, one says that the therapist knows the trauma by the way she feels. This assumes something that is, depending on how you look at it, rather amazing, and also really rather commonplace. And that is that affects inform; they function cognitively. It strikes me that we cannot understand the repetition compulsion unless we assume this, and yet it is a paradox.

At this point I am going to depart from whatever attempts I have made up to now to talk about anything in the real world. I am going to talk instead in terms of myth, allegory, and metaphor. In what follows you will find the metaphor of color and at least four allegories: the burned hand; the philosopher who divides the world in three parts: feelings, thought, and acts; the skier who struggles against his compulsion to fall; and the moralist struggling with love and hate. However, be warned that, as with any myth, you are invited to make it as real as you please.

Compare the range of feelings with the range of colors. Peter Sifneos (1992) uses this analogy when he describes alexithymia as an affective color-blindness. I would like to extend the analogy and say that any psychopathology will necessarily affect, is really defined by, the amount and range of colors with which one sees the world. It is as if the capacity to see the world with a full range of color always exists as a potential but is liable to injury. One color or another may predominate, based on some early experience that etched it out in a determining way. It is as if the perceiving apparatus, having been injured, continues to perceive but fails to develop the capacity to distinguish the old color from new ones.

But the analogy of color suggests something else. Color mediates between the perceiver and that which is perceived. We can say we know the object. It defines the object and makes possible appreciation of it, and yet it is also an internal faculty; it requires a functioning retina, at least, and it has limitations and vulnerabilites.

Think now about an injury to the body, such as a burn. Reparative processes are set into motion. Walter Cannon (1927), in referring to the wisdom of the body, had in mind the capacity of the organism to create and maintain for itself the conditions necessary for life to proceed, that is to say, the self-regulatory, homeostatic mechanisms. One can think of the trauma–injury–healing sequence in this connection. Processes such as inflammation, sequestration, splinting, and scar-tissue formation come to mind. There are instances in which the healing process is fully restorative, but there are also instances in which it somehow miscarries badly and exacerbates the injury, for example in autoimmune disorders.

There are situations where, without sophisticated help, the individual would surely die. Dramatic examples come to the mind of every surgeon, internist, or psychiatrist. And yet for each it is also true that, despite all the modern techniques, in the last analysis one relies on the healing processes within the organism. In fact, the physicianly art consists of fostering, facilitating, and maximizing the inherent thrust toward cure and life. We have to suppose that the basic thrust of life is to repair, restore, heal, and grow, which remains true regardless of whatever metaphor, whatever language, whatever observing instrument we choose to employ.

The basic notions are these: trauma, by definition, is anything that causes injury. Injury, by definition, is anything that necessitates healing. And healing is a process of repair that as a general rule involves pain and dysfunction and requires mobilization of resources. The process, therefore, is costly. It consumes energy, and the organism is constrained to take time off from other enterprises. There is an internal logic, a kind of mathematics, a "wisdom," to all of this that is remarkable. For example, the pain serves as an essential regulatory device. It alerts the organism to the danger of injury (hand too close to the flame), it signals the fact of injury (hand has been burned), and it serves as guardian of the healing processes (the reminder that the hand will require rest and care).

I think you can see the drift of the argument. For pain, read affect. For injury, read injury to the observing instrument, namely the capacity to feel. Psychopathology represents the scar tissue of the injury to the capacity to feel.

Now comes the philosophy, and the going gets a little rough. One of the hallmarks of injury is dysfunction. (The other two are pain and the need to mobilize resources.) We have the injury to the capacity to feel, but what is the dysfunction? Dysfunction of the mind, presumably. Well, what, then, is the mind's function? To act? Let us say to act. The final common pathway of the nervous system is action.

For those of you who have been taught, as I was, to distinguish feeling from thought and affection from cognition, and were further taught that both precede action, there must be something a bit muddled, to say the least, about the notion of the cognitive function of affects. The model is supposed to run from feeling, to thinking, to acting. In health there is a smooth, seamless orchestration of the three. In psychopathology, we have a dysfunctional atrophy or hypertrophy, so that there is, for example, acting out, or "thinking out" (obsessional neurosis), or "feeling out" (hysteria). The more serious kinds of psychopathology include the two major psychoses: thought disorder and affective disorder. Probably equally dysfunctional, although not technically a psychosis, is impulse disorder. This little schema is almost too neat to be genuinely useful.

But feeling, thought, and action cannot really be separated. When one tries to do so, they rush back together, fused, mixed. Each by its very nature includes the other. It is not that affect must somehow be balanced by thought. It is more that we can think only to the extent and degree to which we feel, and vice versa. The reason for discussing the informing function of affects is the curious way in which they *mis*inform in the case of the repetition compulsion. Trauma causes an injury that has the effect of systematically distorting feeling, thinking, and doing, and this *is* the repetition compulsion. But it might be instructive to ponder for a moment why it is that one cannot separate feeling, thinking, and doing.

Any feeling is necessarily connected (however remotely) with an action (actual or potential) and a piece of reality (past or present). Take loneliness, for example. The feeling of loneliness must be something other than simply the past, present, and future state of being alone. It has to include the reality of some significant, important person (currently not present) and an action (leaving, being left). Loneliness assumes its texture, its significance, by contrast to a not-lonely alternative. This contrast can be defined only by reference to another person and to something that one or the other does. Ultimately, it is done by both. For example, the state of being lonely in the midst of people must be something a person actively repeats, as apparently happens in the experience of trauma.

Thoughts, feelings, and acts all inform one another and require one another. Any feeling represents a press (however slight) towards some action, in other words, a wish. However, it requires thought in order to be consummated. Any thought (however abstract) is ultimately defined by the doing of something or other. However, feelings define its relevance. Any act, insofar as it is the product of intent, represents the consummation of a feeling in the context of a judgment. The notion of validity and reality applies to thought and feeling together, but it requires action in order to make discovery of either possible. The Cartesian cleavage between subjective and objective, mental and physical, is a very major confusion. Insofar as the inner and the outer world meet anywhere, they meet, not in the pineal gland, but in the *act*. Feelings are every bit as educable, as shaped by reality, as are thoughts. They have to be; otherwise there would be no possible meaning to psychotherapy.

Competence necessarily weaves together the capacity to think and the capacity to feel. Of the two, the capacity to feel is primary. The Cartesian paraphrase might be: I feel, therefore I think; I feel, therefore I act; I feel, therefore I am. The Cartesian fallacy lies in the quest for "objectivity" somewhere beyond, beneath, outside of, feelings—anywhere, save in the feelings themselves. But ultimately it is the capacity to feel that gives one whatever objectivity one has. Feelings are just as much an avenue of perception, a window onto the world, as are sights, sounds, and touches. They are woven into the texture of external reality in precisely the same way.

Any sensory modality, any sensation at all, can be solipsized. All this does is to demonstrate that objectivity is a task, not something automatically given. But the point is to make use of sensations to tell us something about where we live. Objectivity has to do with the method, not the raw material. The problem of objectifying feelings amounts to the problem of emotional development in general, which faces every individual. A person's feelings define his relationship to the outside world and, most important, to other people. A feeling is the instrumentality, the agency, the vector, the defining energy, of connectedness or attachment. Affects are sufficiently determined by the realities of the world, and by the inner press to act, to make attachments possible. They are sufficiently determined by the inner press to act to make them meaningful. Interruptions of the development of this process appear to have a solipsizing effect.

There is a reality—the same discoverable reality—to both the inner world and the outer world, and one can know the one only by knowing the other. One has both to feel what one knows and know what one feels. Feelings can be known, ultimately, only by objectifying them. And reality is known, ultimately, by scrutiny of what one is aware of.

This process can take place only in a human relationship. This is where the psychoanalytic sense of the word *object* coincides with the philosophical one. The important external reality is the reality of another person about whom one has strong feelings. One needs the relationship to discover what one feels. At one point the feeling reposes on the object: paranoia, let us say. At another point, it reposes on the self: depression. However, each condition in its own way implies that the difference between self and object has not been entirely clinched. And if for any reason the relationship is interrupted, whether actually or in a given emotional context (say the context of trauma), then this is where matters remain. Affective competency in this context is stunted. The feeling is contained, not in the growth potential of the relationship, but in one or another variety of psychopathology.

The capacity to feel involves a complex hierarchy of competencies. One clear example, as Zetzel has shown, is depression. Persons unable to feel depression are seriously handicapped. However difficult, however painful it may be, the capacity to experience depression relieves one of the need for much more constricting and costly mechanisms such as narcissism or paranoia. We know that the person who is capable of depression has been able, at least once in life, to attach and to relate in a way that narcissism or paranoia does not allow. Paranoia, for example, precludes precisely the intimacy that is beyond the capabilities of the individual. The point is not so much that depression is the next rung up on the ladder from paranoia. There are complexities and exceptions, and if we depart too much from the affect itself, we may even be wrong. For the thing that is remarkable is that the affect at a given moment, for a given person, with a given history, in a given situation, is utterly accurate and unerring. It is as if people affectively sculpt for themselves about as much as they can know and deal with at the moment.

Another example of the same thing is the way in which the treatment process discovers the past. There are any number of successive revisions of one's personal past history, based on new levels of affective awareness. There is, therefore, no such thing as a final, objective historical account. However, once one grants this, one discovers an internal logic to the successive unfolding of affective awareness that allows one to say, with as much certainty as is possible anywhere, that this or that must have been real. Here again, one discovers the internal logic, the necessary mathematics, of affective competency.

A third example: a little girl, let us say aged 3 or 4, is sullenly watching her mother breastfeeding a new baby. To the little girl, the new arrival is obviously unwelcome. She points to her mother's breast and says, "It bit me!" What is going on? Let us say we are witnessing a trauma. The baby has taken away the mother's breast, the girl is hurt and wants revenge, a suitable one under the circumstances, but the wish is unacceptable and threatening and is projected. We could, if we want, call her paranoid. But what is important here is something else. And that is that the little girl obviously needs her mother's breast right now in a specific and crucial way. The breast now serves as the receptacle, the container, for something belonging to the little girl that she cannot herself, right now, contain: that is, the wish to injure. This is the only way she can identify and feel her rage. Eventually, if she is to grow, she will need to feel, to own, to contain the wish herself, but right now an essential component of the trauma is that she cannot. She is going to need the breast, over and over again, to project, introject, reproject, reintroject. Melanie Klein (1946) called this phenomenon projective identification, and Otto Kernberg (1975) sees it as underlying the psychopathology of splitting found in the borderline.

For our purposes, let us think of it, not as psychopathology merely, but as the necessary and crucial aspect of the mastery of affects and of reality in general. The breast can become the mother, the mother can become other persons important in the child's later life, only to the extent to which this affective taking-in, giving-out process occurs in an ongoing way. It does not do so if the person is alone. Trauma isolates the individual, and the repetition compulsion is the cry for containment.

In "The role of paradox in the repetition compulsion" (Chapter 1, this volume), I illustrate affective competency through the example of learning to ski. A novice skier seems to favor one ankle. But a doubt occurs. How do we know whether the person actually has had an injury? Might it not be that the problem is somehow "in the mind?" How much in the final analysis is actual trauma, and how much is internal predisposition to trauma? This question is not exactly new. Freud (1917) described the situation as a complemental series: what was not accounted for by trauma was ascribed to internal predisposition. Let us take a moment to trace the notion.

Breuer and Freud (1895) originally proposed a theory emphasizing the trauma. Hysteria, they said, could be explained by a history of actual traumatizing seduction in childhood that left in its wake a pathogenic repressed memory with its quota of strangulated affect. Breuer's concept of the hypnoid state can be thought of as focusing on internal predisposition, whereas Freud at this time emphasized the importance of the reality of the sexual trauma. It is interesting to remember that the trauma, for Freud, was retroactive. He thought, at the time, that childhood was innocent of sexuality, and so the memory set in motion conflict, repression, and symptom formation only with the advent of puberty. The sexual wish, in other words, retroactively informed and defined the earlier situation as a traumatizing one.

The next step was ushered in by the patients whose symptomatology in every way suggested trauma, but in whose case Freud (1914b) was forced, reluctantly at first, to conclude that traumatization must have occurred only in fantasy. The trauma, if we can call it that, becomes a virtual, not an actual one. It occurs via the sexual wish that is present actually, not retroactively, in childhood. The traumatizing reality in the first theory is the parent who actually seduces. In the later theory, the traumatizing reality is the actual wish for the seducing parent.

From this point on, Freud's broadening and elaboration of the concept of trauma begins to blend into the entirety of his psychoanalytic theory. Trauma occurs prehistorically in the form of the history of the race, that is, in inherited, constitutional factors. It occurs at birth. It occurs in the form of childhood traumata leading to fixations. It occurs cumulatively. It occurs in the form of assaults from within, that is, in instinctual anxiety. Broadly speaking, the ego would not develop without the "traumata" delivered to it by the id, the superego, and reality. There is thus a kind of theoretical "complemental series" in the spectrum of Freud's writings. It consists of the fact that the more complex and inclusive the theory becomes, the less possible it is to cast things in terms of trauma versus predisposition.

Freud does, however, deal specifically with the issue of trauma in other writings (e.g., 1914a), and this is because of its intimate connection with the repetition compulsion and with transference. Transference is pinpointed as a necessary, central, and valuable feature of the treatment process. It is a species of the repetition compulsion, and as such it is the vehicle through which the patient relives that which he cannot remember, the trauma.

In *Beyond the Pleasure Principle* (1920), the repetition compulsion is accorded a distinctive position: it is the closest glimpse we have of the otherwise silent operation of the death instinct. Freud describes the painful repetition of the trauma as truly compulsive, as "daemonic." It goes beyond any possible pleasure, beyond even the attempt to repeat in the service of active mastery. It can be understood only as the attempt to restore the earliest state of affairs. Trauma overwhelms the ego's capacity to respond at the time and therefore leaves a residue of tension that can be bound and later discharged only by successive repetition. This bespeaks a return not to a constant, usable quantity of tension in the service of reality testing (i.e., the ego, the constancy principle), but rather the wish for total absence of tension (the nirvana principle, death). It is as if, insofar as the experience of trauma is repeated, the individual expresses a total loss of resources, a wish to die.

The implications of all of this for life in general, and the treatment process in particular, are hardly optimistic. Freud himself drew back at this point: "But let us pause for a moment and reflect. It cannot be so" (p. 39). He then reminds himself, and us, of the force of life, of Eros, of love. And so what emerges is the now familiar antithesis between Eros and Thanatos, Life and

Death, Love and Hate. Every human being must necessarily experience the lifelong struggle between these two forces. Trauma is simply the name, specific to the individual, of the way in which the struggle is repeated.

But there is still a problem. It is the same one we had on the ski slope. The thrust of the skiing analogy was that it might be possible to cast the entire matter in terms of the mathematics of competence. But can we? How are we to understand the intransigence of the residual pockets of incompetence, the malignant repetitions of trauma, the severity of psychopathology? My reading of Freud is that, for him, this is something beyond mathematics, beyond the simple repeating of things not yet solved. The repetition compulsion is "daemonic." At the moment the individual is caught up in it, he is in the grips of the fundamental biological return of all living substance toward death. The question is, how much is this a metaphorical description of what one feels when one repeats, and how much is it the actual state of affairs? Is Freud talking about the Snow Snake that makes skiers fall, or do we really, in some profound sense, cease to live when we repeat?

Let me suggest, to begin with, that we take the notion of the death wish quite seriously. It is not obviously wrong. One usually hears that aggression is the basic instinct, but that the idea of a death wish is mystical, unprovable. But this won't do. Freud's conception is a deeper one. A death wish amounts to a wish for death, whether one's own or somebody else's. Hate is the death wish, and love and hate lie at the very core of what trauma is all about. Insofar as one loves, one lives. Insofar as one hates, one dies. Murder and suicide are basically equivalent. Suicide is a supremely hostile, aggressive act, and murder is in the final analysis self-destructive. A quote from Winnicott (1958) comes to mind: "in some specific setting, of which the patient is unaware, hate is more powerful than love" (p. 20). Winnicott was discussing the sense of guilt, but could these words not also serve as the definition of trauma in general, of repetition in general, of pychopathology in general?

Insofar as one is traumatized, insofar as one repeats the past, insofar as one hates, to that extent one murders time, does not choose, does not act, does not live. In other words, trauma, the repetition compulsion, the wish to kill, illness, and the sapping of the energies of life are intimately bound together.

Sex and aggression are not the same as love and hate. Sexuality can be used in the service of love. It can also be used in the service of hate. This is clearly so in the case of rape. It also occurs, as Stoller (1974) has shown, in a somewhat more muted way with perversions in general. In fact, to whatever degree a person cannot use sexuality in the service of love, this is because it has become entrained in the service of hate. Similarly, aggression can be used in the service of either love or hate. The question of how much of one's aggressive energies are used in the service of love, activity, and the tasks of life on the one hand, and how much in the service of hate on the other, is probably one that cannot be decided in advance. It is decided by the events of life—in some measure, that is to say, by trauma. We have already seen that for a variety of reasons there is no such thing as life without trauma. But it is also clear that there are real differences in the degree and the kind of injuries that an individual sustains, and that hate is related in a very real way to those injuries. Hate occurs in response to an injury to the self. It is a species of pain, except that, because it is the wish to injure, kill, and destroy, it can, like autoimmune disease, become an illness itself. The education and transformation of affects, leading to competence, amounts to the transformation of wishes. Every stage of life has its own version of the struggle between the wish to kill and the yearning for attachment. Every variety of psychopathology can be thought of as one particular instance in a long series of compromise solutions to the problems of violence versus intimacy. The trauma is capable of inflicting injury, ultimately, because urgency is given to the sorts of wishes that threaten the fabric of life. The wish to kill would not be traumatizing to the person who has no attachment to that which he wishes to kill. But, in fact, this never happens. How is it possible to hate the loved and loving object, and live?

What has to happen, of course, is that one must discover a situation, a relationship, where there is a familiar urgency to the destructive wish, but where, in fact, other wishes are possible. Containment amounts to holding in hand both the wishes and their consequences, as possibilities, against the time when there can be a real choice. To choose not to kill is a different matter from the control of the wish to kill. The more profound wish is the wish to love, but it must be discovered, and the hate is on loan against the time when the healing can occur.

But we now have to remember: all of this was intended as myth, metaphor, and allegory. We took Freud seriously, but we still have the death wish. Is it real, or is it a myth? What about love? Is that real, or is it a moral allegory? The answer, of course, can come only from the feelings themselves. Whatever is true is so because of what one already feels, knows, and does. The death wish is real, exists, for the person who feels hate. And we all do. And love exists insofar as we can feel it.

What we have just done is to retrace the same steps in terms of trauma and the wish to destroy as did Freud originally in terms of trauma and the sexual wish. One theory is a theory of injury from the outside, in which the hate retroactively informs the trauma. We then discover that the injury can be internal, the actuality of the wish for injury. And we then see that the theoretical complemental series applies here as well. The more you get into it, the more difficult it is to say what is trauma and what is predisposition, what is outside and what is inside. It begins to dawn on us that this is the way things happen when there has been trauma. The capacity to know clearly what one feels, what is versus what was, what is inside versus what is outside, can occur only when there has been healing and growth. One of the features of trauma is that the trauma itself cannot at the time be fully felt and known, let alone acted upon. It takes healing to know the injury. And healing of the injury requires, as does emotional growth itself, the containment provided by human relationships.

It is possible to show, as Freud did first in terms of the sexual wish, that hate energizes virtually every thought, feeling, and action, every trauma. Hate and love are therefore paradigms of the capacity to feel. They demonstrate the manner in which any feeling, any wish, is discoverable and defines reality. Discovery occurs only in a relationship, and the feelings become the defining reality of the relationship. The capacity to feel is itself a discoverable competency, a faculty subject to development, growth, and life, as well as to trauma, injury, and death. But the capacity to feel is the window to life.

Trauma to the psyche, like trauma to the body, creates damage that requires repair. The bonds of connectedness, of attachment, must be created anew. And this means, necessarily, the recapitulation in some measure of the ways those bonds were woven to begin with, with all the early uncertainties of inner and outer reality. The treatment process discovers the feelings and the injury to them. The trauma represents a crisis in which there is either mastery and growth, or a closing off of the development of competence that necessitates the repetition of the defining feeling. The affect sculpts out exactly the problem of relatedness that has not yet been solved. Reality, therefore, is determined by what one can feel.

But let me finish the allegory. One needs the myth until one knows the feeling. The final allegory is love. Love is a competence. More exactly, love is the final competence. One is competent only to the extent and to the degree that one can love. The capacity to love is the capacity to create, nurture, and cherish life, and competence involves the capacity to feel as wishes those actions that in reality are fostering of life. Containment and love are one and the same.

REFERENCES

Anscombe, R. (1981). Philosophical critique of Schafer's action language. *International Journal of Psycho-Analysis* 62:225–247.

Breuer, J. and Freud, S. (1895). Studies on hysteria. *Standard Edition* 2.

Cannon, W. B. (1927). The James–Lange theory of emotion: a critical examination and an alternative theory. *American Journal of Psychology* 39:106–124.

Erikson, K. T. (1976). *Everything in its Path: Destruction of the Community in the Buffalo Creek Flood.* New York: Simon & Schuster.

Freud, S. (1914a). Remembering, repeating, and working-through. *Standard Edition* 12:147–156.

——— (1914b). On the history of the psycho-analytic movement. *Standard Edition* 14:3–66.

——— (1917). Introductory Lectures on Psycho-Analysis. *Standard Edition* 16.

——— (1920). Beyond the Pleasure Principle. *Standard Edition* 18:3–64.

Haley, S. (1974). When the patient reports atrocities. *Archives of General Psychiatry* 30:191–196.

Kernberg, O. (1975). *Borderline Conditions and Pathological Narcissism.* New York: Jason Aronson.

Klein, M. (1946). Notes on some schizoid mechanisms. *International Journal of Psycho-Analysis* 27:99–110.

Russell, P. (1975). The theory of the crunch. Unpublished manuscript.

——— (1976). Beyond the wish. Unpublished manuscript.

Sifneos, P. (1992). *Short Term Anxiety Provoking Psychotherapy. A Treatment Manual.* New York: Basic Books.

Stoller, R. J. (1974). Hostility and mystery in perversion. *International Journal of Psycho-Analysis* 55:425–438.

Winnicott, D. W. (1958). Psycho-analysis and the sense of guilt. In *The Maturational Processes and the Facilitating Environment*, pp. 15–28. New York: International Universities Press.

THREE

LETTING THE PARADOX TEACH US

Stephen A. Mitchell, Ph.D.

I first began to get to know analysts and those interested in becoming analysts outside of New York City in the mid-1980s, through what was then called the local chapters movement of Division 39 of the American Psychological Association. Sparked by the establishment of the Colorado Center in Denver, interested groups were forming in many major cities, including Boston, Chicago, Washington, Toronto, San Francisco, Oklahoma City, and Seattle. Although participants in these groups reflected the entire spectrum of theoretical orientations, the majority had been most influenced by the major post-classical authors: Sullivan, Fairbairn, Winnicott, Loewald, and Kohut.

The group from Boston was generally like the others in most respects, but in the creative papers they began producing, one odd detail emerged. They all tended to cite, often more than the other major authors whose work I knew well, a man named Paul Russell, with whom I was not familiar. As the citations and quotations accumulated, I began to get a sense of Russell's concerns and contributions, but then I encountered a further oddity: these papers that had such a big impact on this new generation of clinicians and theorists, these papers of Russell's, were all unpublished. Over the years I was able to obtain some of the manuscripts myself, so as to be able to sample the richness of Russell's thought first-hand. And I met him briefly, sharing a panel in Boston with him shortly before his death. I began to develop a sense of this man as an extraordinary teacher. I could see why those who had studied with him cited him so frequently, because his thinking seemed to have had such a fecund, richly resonating impact on the multiple paths that were emerging from this younger generation of psychoanalytic thinkers from Boston. I am therefore pleased to have been invited to participate in this project of bringing Russell's work to the attention of the wider audience it so clearly deserves.

However, I find that writing about Russell's papers is not easy. His writing is extraordinarily lucid, both intricate and simple, complex and epigrammatic, with a no-frills, distilled wisdom. He writes about what seems most central to clinical work and human suffering and growth. He boils down elaborate lines of theorizing to basic concepts and principles, positioning and repositioning them in relation to each other, exploring each important facet and nuance in turn, working and reworking the same central, dense, paradoxical phenomena. It is hard to know what else one would want to say. So what seems most appropriate for me on this occasion is to pull out of the two papers of Russell's that are reproduced here the concepts that are most provocative for me and to develop some of my associations to them. I find that my associations generally take the form of an appreciation of Russell's way of conceptualizing and depicting key issues, and I often find myself exploring links to other writers, past and present. The intent here is not so much to present an organized commentary on Russell's ideas as to illustrate the ways in which he alerts us to the hub of major themes of post-classical psychoanalytic thought.

Like Fairbairn, Russell places painful repetition at the center of our clinical concerns: psychopathology *is* the repetition compulsion. I like the way he uses Freud's descriptive clinical genius without being encumbered by Freud's metapsychological systems. Russell draws on Kuhn to demonstrate the ways in which old systems are broken apart by the anomalous; and there *is* always an anomalous, he suggests, because systems establish continuity and consistency partly through exclusion. (Here Russell sounds like Foucault, minus the obscurity.) And oddly enough, the anomalous, the excluded, for Freud's hedonic metapsychology, was always painful repetition: nightmares, masochism, fate neurosis, battle, and other traumatic neuroses. Freud couldn't explain these, to his own satisfaction, within the confines of the pleasure principle, but it was his genius to hold onto and continue to grapple with what he couldn't satisfactorily explain. Russell explores repetition from many angles: as an effort at mastery through familiarity and reversal (like Freud and the ego psychologists); as an attempt to continue an interrupted relationship (like Fairbairn); as an abortive attempt at self-healing (like Winnicott); as maturational impairment (like contemporary developmental theorists); as a distorted form of, or replacement for, memory (somewhat like Loewald); as interpersonal incompetence (like Levenson). By exploring each facet of repetition in turn, Russell manages to be simple and close to clinical experience without being reductive.

Russell calls our attention to the central dialectic in human growth between continuity and change. (This theme has been richly developed in the recent papers of Philip Bromberg, e.g.,

1993.) Growth stops abruptly at points where any change threatens to destroy continuity. Continuity is supplied through human relationship. Relationships stop growing when they cannot contain important wishes. Affects and cognition are inseparable from each other, and embedded in affects are wishes. (This theme has been developed extensively by Spezzano 1993.) The conflict between maintaining the continuity of the relationship and expressing the wish is no real choice at all: continuity always wins, but disguised, healing wishes perpetually push through. These wishes *are* psychopathology. Russell reminds us that Freud's great achievement was not in the specific wishes (sex and aggression) he privileged, but in opening up the exploration of the clash between wishes in general and continuity of relationship. (For a similar argument, see Greenberg 1991.)

Russell brings all this together with great clarity and succintness. Sometimes, he suggests, clinical work goes smoothly, and we take these rarities as the model. But that is very misleading. Ordinarily, as Russell demonstrates with a persuasiveness by which he might be demonstrating why day must follow night, the patient and the analyst are, necessarily, in for a hard time. In other writings, he aptly terms this hard time "the crunch." The patient is convinced that the expression of the anomalous wish is not containable within the relationship. He longs for something different but is certain that forbidden wishes will obliterate whatever modicum of security he has been able to maintain. The analyst, too, wants things both to remain the same and to change. The analyst's empathy is not enough; his passion is necessary as well (Russell calls it the analyst's "urgency").

Part of what is impressive about Russell's descriptions of the transference–countertransference enmeshments at the core of the analytic process is the way he simply takes for granted, and writes about with great obviousness, some of the most controversial of contemporary notions about the analytic process. Two of the most important are the following.

First, the threat to the analytic relationship is not simply a transferential displacement from the past; it is really happening in the here and now. The patient needs the analyst to feel and do things that the analyst is frightened to feel and do. The patient needs the analyst to occupy two, mutually exclusive, places at the same time. The analyst wants both to keep doing what he has always done and to participate in a kind of change that requires him to find something different to do. All this cannot be simply understood as a displaced reality from a different time; it is real now, and significant change can occur only if it is lived through by both parties in the here and now. A patient of mine recently expressed these challenges by explaining that the alternatives we had been exploring seemed hard for her to avail herself of. She had trouble imagining that I or other important people in her life could possibly tolerate her expression of her own, heretofore unexpressed, needs. And she had trouble imagining that she could operate differently and still remain herself.

A second controversial principle that Russell writes about with great lucidity is the centrality of the affective exchange between patient and analyst. The ability to preserve the relationship while sustaining wishes that are felt to be obliterative is key to the patient's growth, he suggests. For the patient to take that leap of faith, the analyst must struggle through his own resistances to feeling what must be felt. This cannot be faked. Technique (as it is ordinarily talked about) will not do. The analyst's presence with the patient as the latter straddles old and new does not necessarily have to be spoken, but, Russell suggests, it must be felt. It cannot be postured. Thus, Russell seems to imply, affects are palpably knowable; the analyst must come to know what the patient feels, and the patient will inevitably know what the analyst feels. It is only through negotiation between the two parties, opening up a path that never existed before, that continuity and change, the old and the new, relationship and growth, become simultaneous possibilities.

Some of Russell's richest descriptions of the analytic process entail his use of the concept of paradox to depict the logical structure of "the crunch," through which thicket the analysand and analyst must negotiate a path. Stuart Pizer (1998) has elaborated and illustrated the centrality of the negotiation of paradox, and, although they did not use the term *paradox*, some of my favorite accounts of the analytic process have grappled with the same seeming impossibility that Russell portrays. Thus Fairbairn (1952) suggests that the patient cannot possibly give up his adhesive attachment to bad objects unless he has confidence in the possibility of the analyst as a new object. But the patient cannot possibly believe in the analyst as a new object unless he renounces his attachment to his old objects. Similarly, Lawrence Friedman (1988) has pointed out that the transferential importance the patient attributes to the analyst is what imparts power to interpretations, yet the most important interpretations are those that systematically dismantle the analyst's transferential significance. Similarly, Russell's depictions of "the crunch" provide a vivid addition to these orienting and inspirational accounts of the leap of faith required of both participants in the analytic process. As Russell puts it, "we are negotiating . . . something that has never happened before, namely the experience of loss and detachment in the presence of attachment, of containment" (this volume, p. 16).

Russell wants us to learn, as readers, analysts, and patients, from sustaining the tensions inherent in paradoxes. Emmanuel

Letting the Paradox Teach Us

Ghent (1992) has suggested that sometimes the sustaining and exploration of paradox reveals the paradox to be only apparent, concealing an underlying defensive process. But for Russell, paradoxes arise when the patient pushes for the anomalous in the context of the familiar, for change in the context of continuity. "A paradox is *something that the coherence and consistency of the entire rest of the system require to be both true and not true, a contradiction from which there is no escape without the destruction of the system*" (this volume, p. 15). Engaging and sustaining the paradox blows the old system apart, just enough, for some new organization to emerge.

But Russell also wants us to appreciate the paradoxical nature of human growth in more general terms, the processes that make possible the emergence of the new from the old, the present from the perpetual past, externality from projections, agency from embeddedness. He points to four essential paradoxes in the growth of human feeling by posing four seemingly unanswerable questions: "Is this me, or is this you? Did I do this, or was it done to me? Is this now, or was it then? Can I choose what I feel?" (p. 8). In his discussion of these questions, I found Russell uncharacteristically elusive. "What is to become of these ambiguities?" I found myself wondering. At some points Russell seems to suggest that they will be resolved as each traumatic repetition is lived through, as the old organization cracks under the pressure the paradoxes generate and a new organization emerges. At other points Russell seems to be suggesting that these essential paradoxes are inherent in human experience and necessarily remain. But how?

It is here that I found it useful to connect Russell's depiction of essential paradoxes with Loewald's (1980) notion of a perpetual tension between primary process and secondary process as ongoing organizations through which experience is generated. The distinctions between me and you, activity and passivity, now and then are logical distinctions belonging to what Loewald would consider secondary process. All these distinctions, he argues, are not givens but rather are constructions that appear as developmental achievements. In our processing of our earliest experiences and in moments of great affective intensity and emotional trauma, experience is organized through a primary process in which the secondary-process distinctions do not operate. Because on a primary-process level minds are permeable, interactions are co-constructed, and time is not linear but simultaneous, separation into the neat categories of secondary process (me/you, then/now, acting/acted upon) can never be complete. On a primary-process level, the contradictions that generate the paradoxes disappear because their incompatible categories dissolve.

In Loewald's way of thinking, we live simultaneously on two levels of mental organization, a secondary process in which dichotomous distinctions are necessary for adaptively and effectively negotiating the world, and a primary process in which we are in touch with and part of an original, dense unity where there are no neat categories to sort things out. In his final book, Loewald (1988) goes to some length to distinguish his account of these matters from the closely related contributions of Winnicott. Although the latter sees great significance and value in primary-process kinds of experiences (subjective omnipotence, transitional experiencing, and the like), he regards them as creative illusions, enriching the more objective world of conventional reality. Loewald stresses that primary process and secondary process are two alternative forms of organizing experience. Both are equally real; there is no illusion involved. (For an exploration of this contrast between Loewald and Winnicott, see Mitchell 1999.) It is that very doubleness of experience, simultaneously organized on two different levels with two different organizational structures, that builds paradox necessarily into the very nature of human experience. In poignant emotional moments, it is neither possible nor necessary to sort out me from you. At points of personal growth and transcendence, it is neither possible nor helpful to distinguish what was done to me from what I generated myself. In the richest affective experiences, it is neither possible nor enriching to distinguish between now and then.

For me, Loewald's contributions illuminate Russell's claim that paradox is essential to growth. In Russell's sense, old systems that we need for continuity must break apart in the change that is essential to real living. In Loewald's sense, the dense affective unities of primary-process organization ensure both that nothing ever completely changes and that all our transitory secondary-process categories will be perpetually broken up by the flux of unconscious experience. Both Loewald and Russell agree that we serve our patients best when we find new ways of helping them sustain these paradoxical tensions.

Part of what I value most about Russell's writings is that he is unafraid to acknowledge that we will never fully account for the mystery of human change. Theorists in artificial intelligence tell us that our minds are self-programming programs, that we grow in "crazy loops" in which we use our prior organizational schemes to bootstrap ourselves into new organizational schemes. We can describe that process, but nobody really understands how it actually works. Psychoanalysts can help generate and participate in emotional contexts in which deeply significant growth might take place. But each situation is different, each is custom designed, and we can never know for sure when growth will occur. The best we can do, as Russell suggests, is to try to stay as open as possible to letting the paradoxes teach us.

REFERENCES

Bromberg, P. M. (1993). Shadow and substance. *Psychoanalytic Psychology* 10(2):147–168.

Fairbairn, R. W. D. (1952). *An Object-Relations Theory of the Personality*. New York: Basic Books.

Friedman, L. (1988). *The Anatomy of Psychotherapy*. Hillsdale, NJ: Analytic Press.

Ghent, E. (1992). Process and paradox. *Psychoanalytic Dialogues* 2(4):135–160.

Greenberg, J. (1991). *Oedipus and Beyond*. Cambridge, MA: Harvard University Press.

Levenson, E. (1983). *The Ambiguity of Change: An Inquiry into the Nature of Psychoanalytic Reality*. New York: Basic Books.

Loewald, H. (1980). *Papers on Psychoanalysis*. New Haven: Yale University Press.

——— (1988). *Sublimation*. New Haven: Yale University Press.

Mitchell, S. A. (1999). From ghosts to ancestors: the psychoanalytic vision of Hans Loewald. *Psychoanalytic Dialogues* 9 (in press).

Pizer, S. A. (1998). *Negotiation of Paradox in Psychoanalysis*. Hillsdale, NJ: Analytic Press.

Spezzano, C. (1993). *Affects in Psychoanalysis*. Hillsdale, NJ: Analytic Press.

FOUR

WINDOWS OPENED AND CLOSED: REPETITION AND DEFICIT IN THE NEGOTIATION OF AFFECT

Arnold H. Modell, M.D.

Paul Russell was one of the most original and gifted contributors to psychiatry and psychoanalysis. Unfortunately this fact was known only to the limited circle of his students and friends who read his unpublished manuscripts. It is sad and ironic that only after his death will his work receive the attention that it deserves.

At a symposium in Boston in 1985, I discussed an earlier draft of "The role of paradox in the repetition compulsion." I would judge this paper today, as I did then, to be a classic. Paul had the poet's gift of identifying timeless human predicaments. Nevertheless, while our predicaments may remain timeless, even in the relatively short time since this study was presented there have been changes within the field of psychoanalysis as well as advances within neurobiology and infant research that have implications for the two papers published here. I am sure that Paul would have welcomed these changes and would have incorporated them into his work.

Within the culture of psychoanalysis there is today an altered attitude toward what might be called the authority of the past. The significance of the past that Freud attributed to the repetition compulsion has been overshadowed by the current focus upon intersubjectivity, a process that, on first inspection, appears to operate in the here and now. "The role of paradox in the repetition compulsion" can be seen as a corrective to what may be a shallow understanding of the importance of the here and now. For the present is always shadowed by the past. I would underline the significance of what Paul emphasized, namely the paradox of our experience of time. This paradox was first noted in the fourth century by Saint Augustine: "Thus my childhood, which now is not, is in time past, which now is not: but now when I recall its image, and tell of it, I behold it in the present, because it is still in my memory. Yet it might be properly said there be three times: a present of things past, a present of things present, and a present of things future" (p. 265). As Hans Loewald (1980) said, "the present does not change the past but it changes that past which the patient carries within as living history" (p. 144). It is a cause for wonder that experiences within the analytic relationship, in real time, can alter affective memories of the past.

I am in nearly complete agreement with both of these papers. What I shall do is to present my own understanding of the repetition compulsion, which is, I believe quite consistent with Russell's views but seen from a somewhat different perspective. However I have one difference with Paul Russell regarding the repetition compulsion, in that I do not attribute it, as Freud did, to the death instinct. I believe that the repetition compulsion can be fully understood as an aspect of memory without recourse to the concept of instinct. Yet it is hard to know how seriously Russell believed in Freud's death instinct, for in "The role of paradox in the repetition compulsion" he treats it as if it were a romantic metaphor.

I would underline the importance of Paul's view that the repetition compulsion "would seem to be two things. One is the nucleus of an organized system of affective incompetence, a dysfunctional feeling system. It is also an attempt to continue an interrupted relationship in the service of . . . emotional growth" (this volume, p. 7). And in "Trauma and the cognitive function of affects" we read that "[t]houghts, feelings, and acts all inform one another and require one another" (p. 35). I would add memory to this statement, so that it would read: "Thoughts, feelings, memory, and acts all inform one another and require one another." I would further paraphrase this assertion to state that memory, affects, and metaphor form a synergistic system.

Our understanding of the repetition compulsion has been enlarged by recent research in the area of memory and metaphor. I am referring to advances in linguistics (Lakoff 1987) that have redefined metaphor and especially to the revolutionary theory of memory proposed by the Nobel laureate Gerald Edelman (1989). Edelman's theory of memory is revolutionary in that he proposes that memory is both categorical and retranscriptive. This represents a sharp break with the traditional idea of memory as a storage system from which items are retrieved. Memory is not a process of retrieval from some static memory bank, because the brain's memory is not like that of the long-term memory of a computer. What the brain stores is not simply isomorphic with perception; experiential memory is actively selective in accordance with past memorial categories. Experiential memory exists as a latent potential that can be revived as an actual memory if current inputs, specifically metonymic associations (the part substituting for the whole) re-evoke the original experience.

I view the repetition compulsion as the activation, through metonymic associations, of old affect categories (Modell 1990).

Using Edelman's theory of memory, I have introduced the term *affect category* to refer to the fact that salient affective memories are stored as potential categories that are evoked when there is a metaphoric correspondence between those affective memories of the past and current perception. What is stored in memory is not a replica of an event but the potential to refind the category of which the event is a member. In this way memory, affects, and metaphor form a synergistic system. As Paul indicates, action is an important component of this system. Edelman, too, proposed that action is an essential component of memory. Cognition is a dynamic process of interaction with the environment, and memory can be considered as a form of cognition. The older view that contrasted a passive sensory system with an active motor system is entirely incorrect (Thelen and Smith 1994). The compulsion to repeat, therefore, represents a compulsion to seek a perceptual identity between present and past objects.

The fact that some patients are unconsciously motivated to evoke in the analyst the very same noxious affective responses that they have experienced in the past from salient others may be understood as an aspect of memory actively aiding cognition. It is adaptive to be vigilant against past dangers. Through affective action the individual can transform the human environment to correspond to that of the past. Postulating that affects have a cognitive task to perform, Paul describes this process as affect training. His formulation of affect training is highly original, but I believe that he is conflating two different processes that sometimes appear together and sometimes do not. For affect training in the therapeutic setup may represent the need to recontextualize or retranscribe old affect categories, or it may represent a developmental deficit in affect regulation. This distinction is meaningful in that different therapeutic processes are involved.

One process may be described as affect recategorization. This occurs when transference repetition becomes transference resolution. A very different process is at work when there has been a developmental deficit in affect regulation. The concept of disorders in affect regulation was not well understood when Paul wrote these papers. We are now better able to understand affect regulation as a result of the contribution of psychoanalytic infant observation. In 1985 infant research was just beginning to emerge as a discipline. By now, however, infant researchers have described in great detail the normative process of mutual affect regulation between caretaker and infant (Schore 1994, Stern 1985). Winnicott's aphorism that there is no such thing as an infant is an accurate observation of the brain as well as the mind, in that the infant's homeostatic systems require the presence of the caretaker. In order for children to develop a capacity for affect regulation, their mothers must be affectively responsive to them and in turn be able to contain and tolerate their children's affective responses. If the maternal environment is not adequate in this regard, a variety of difficulties may ensue. Affect dysregulation may take many forms: affective experiences may be externalized as if the affects were not generated within the self but had as their source some process outside of the self, or the individual may not be able to differentiate or identify different affective experiences, or the individual may feel flooded and overwhelmed by intense feeling and hence avoid close human contact. These are people who cannot stand being emotionally touched. In some cases intense feelings such as sexual arousal may lead to the fear that the self will disintegrate. It is evident that affect dysregulation, a developmental deficit, persists into adult life.

When Paul describes affect training, it is not clear whether that training is required because of a developmental deficit or because of a need to recreate the past in real time (what we ordinarily think of as the effects of the repetition compulsion). The repetition compulsion is universal. But developmental deficits are not universal, so that all those who are driven by a need to repeat the past will not necessarily have also suffered from a developmental deficit of affect regulation.

Transference repetition is understood as an instance of the repetition compulsion and can be thought of as a frozen metaphor in which some aspect of the analyst, in the here and now, will trigger a metonymic association evoking an old affect category. Consequently, the current scene is experienced as an identical metaphoric fit with that of the past. From this point of view, the aim of psychoanalysis is to transform the frozen metaphor into a fluid metaphor in which there is the simultaneous experience of similarity and difference. In general this process is described as resolving the transference. We know that this is accomplished by a variety of means, including interpretation, which, apart from its content, is itself a message: "I am not X, Y, or Z." For interpretations to be effective they must be delivered at the point of the analysand's emotional intensity, but the analysand must also be able to perceive that the analyst's affective response is different from that of X, Y, or Z.

This could be described as a kind of affect training, but it is a different process from that of repairing a developmental deficit. Paul uses the metaphor of learning to ski as an analogy to affect training. In learning to ski the novice imitates and borrows the expert's technique. It is a process of learning similar to what Vygotsky described when the less competent individual learns from the more competent: "The tutor or the aiding peer serves the learner as a vicarious form of consciousness until such time as the learner is able to master his own actions through his own consciousness" (quoted in Modell 1990, p. 96). The concept of vicariously borrowing the tutor's more advanced form of consciousness seems to me to be central to what Paul Russell describes as learning to be affectively competent. Infant researchers such as Edward Tronick (1997) believe that the infant requires the mother's more complex consciousness for homeostasis. Thus, as analysts, we are attempting to repeat a process that had its origins in the first and second years of life. The patient requires that our states of consciousness be such that we can both tolerate intense affects and identify them as our own without having to resort to projection and externalization. Paul movingly describes the traumatizing effects of failures of containment.

We also know from infant research that there are crucial windows of developmental opportunity that remain open for a period of time and then close. I suspect that this is true with regard to affect regulation. With some patients affect retraining can be accomplished in adult life, but this is analogous to the difficulty one has in acquiring a new language in later life.

In these papers there is a promise of a profound and brilliant re-examination of our assumptions regarding affects. Russell had an exquisite sensitivity to the meaning of trauma both to the one who had been traumatized and to the therapist listening to the retelling of the trauma. For Russell, the Cartesian distinction between thinking and feeling made no sense at all. He viewed affects, no less than thought, as a way of knowing the world and believed that those who have been traumatized experience a different logic. We are given a glimpse of a powerful new theory of affects but then are saddened by the realization that Paul Russell was not able to complete this work.

REFERENCES

Augustine. *Confessions*, trans. E. B. Pusey. London: Dent, 1939.

Edelman, G. M. (1989). *The Remembered Present*. New York: Basic Books.

Lakoff, G. (1987). *Women, Fire, and Dangerous Things*. Chicago: University of Chicago Press.

Loewald, H. (1980). *Papers on Psychoanalysis*. New Haven: Yale University Press.

Modell, A. (1990). *Other Times, Other Realities*. Cambridge, MA: Harvard University Press.

Schore, A. N. (1994). *Affect Regulation and the Origin of the Self*. Hillsdale, NJ: Lawrence Erlbaum.

Stern, D. (1985). *The Interpersonal World of the Infant*. New York: Basic Books.

Thelen, E. and Smith, L. (1994). *A Dynamic Systems Approach to the Development of Cognition and Action*. Cambridge, MA: MIT Press.

Tronick, E. (1997). Dyadically expanded states of consciousness and the process of therapeutic change. Unpublished paper.

FIVE

DIFFERENTIATING THE REPETITION COMPULSION FROM TRAUMA THROUGH THE LENS OF TOMKINS'S SCRIPT THEORY: A RESPONSE TO RUSSELL

E. Virginia Demos, Ed. D.

I am very grateful for the invitation to respond to these two papers by Paul Russell, for they have provided me the opportunity to think through, tease out, and articulate how my particular stance differs from my reading of Russell's stance. Both of us place affect and affect dynamics at the center of our understanding of psychopathology and treatment. But while I do not fit comfortably into any particular camp, he seems to have clearly placed himself in the relational or interpersonalist camp. So to some extent our differences consist of the relative importance we would place on the relationship, both in development and in the treatment setting. I would like to embrace the powerful role of interpersonal experience, while at the same time holding onto the importance of intrapsychic dynamics.

Indeed, Russell seems to be doing this when he writes about affect within the therapeutic situation, for example the need for the therapist to be able to stay with, endure, and contain the painful affects of the patient if healing is to occur; the unerring accuracy of the patient's feelings; and the paradox of the therapeutic setting in which the very safety that is created brings with it the threat of disruption through repetition in the transference. I find his writings most eloquent and compelling when he discusses the crisis moments in therapy when the repetition compulsion is fully activated. He articulates quite beautifully how, at such moments, the therapist's affective availability can allow her to enter into the patient's affective world enough so that she is able to understand more accurately the patient's experience and to offer some form of mastery and relief through containment and connection.

But when Russell steps back from the affective heat in the therapeutic work and begins to speak more generally about the repetition compulsion, the healing process, affects, and the role of relationships, he and I begin to part company. The reader may well ask: What difference does it make what his theory is, if his therapeutic writings and presumably his therapeutic work are useful and make sense? Or to phrase the question somewhat differently: Does the relationship between one's theories and the way one works with patients matter? Setting aside for another time the question of the nature of this relationship and a discussion of all the possible ways in which one's theories or beliefs might affect one's therapeutic work, I would like to suggest the following. If we accept that thought and feeling and action are connected in complex and subtle ways, then the interplay between one's theories and one's stance toward patients *must* be important. This paper, therefore, is an effort to sort out and clarify a slightly different perspective that gives full rein to both intrapsychic and interpersonal phenomena as it explores affects, psychopathology, the repetition compulsion,

Differentiating the Repetition Compulsion

healing, and relationships in development and in the therapeutic setting. Whether this conceptual shift will lead to a shift in therapeutic work will be left to the reader to decide and experience, or to a later opportunity when case material could be addressed from different perspectives.

I want to begin with the "healing process" and with Russell's choice of physical injury as an analogy to "psychic injury." Analogies are always seductive, and they are useful only as long as they help us see things about a phenomenon that we might not have fully appreciated without their help. The model of physical injury and a healing process that produces a scar has perhaps grown out of psychiatry's historical connection to the field of medicine. It focuses our attention on aspects of a process that include pain, a marshaling of resources and energy that may be costly to the organism, and a time-consuming rebuilding of tissue. But beyond these aspects, the analogy to psychic injury and healing breaks down because the nature of the two "healing" processes is profoundly different. The healing of injured tissue is governed by physiological processes that are more or less automatic and predictable. For although healing of tissue can be delayed or complicated by repeated injury and/or by infection, it cannot be stopped (except by death or disease), and its progression and outcome (a scar) fall within a very limited range of possible variations.

But as soon as one enters the realm of psychological "injury" and "healing," which are governed primarily by psychological processes, individual variation predominates, and the number of relevant and possible active elements increases radically. The vicissitudes of relationships, the range and varying intensity of affects, the pacing and nature of environmental events, the changing availability of consciousness, and the possibility of choices, as well as many other elements, are all involved. Thus the psychological "healing" process, its progression (which can include a complete cessation of "healing"), and its outcome are highly unpredictable and may involve a continuous process of change and reworking, such that an endpoint or outcome comparable to a scar might not exist or might be extremely difficult to determine. Indeed, these psychological processes are so different that the term *healing* may not be the most appropriate descriptor. Certainly physiological processes are complex and dynamic, but the degrees of freedom are few when compared to the degrees of freedom in psychological processes. This increase in indeterminacy in the psychological realm is directly linked to the role of consciousness and the possibility of choice, as well as to the nature of affect, cognition, and perception and their interrelationships in all efforts to manage psychological pain.

What, then, can be meant by the phrase "psychic injury"? Russell uses the term *trauma* to describe psychic injury, suggesting that every empathic break is experienced as a trauma and that the essence of the trauma is the loss of the relationship. I am perplexed and confused by this use of the term *trauma*. Does he mean to suggest that all experiences of negative affect, regardless of which negative affects and at what intensities, are equally injurious and traumatic? Or is he suggesting that the human psyche, on its own, is so fragile it cannot tolerate even the slightest anxiety or lack of empathic attunement? Either way, such a conceptualization imposes an impossible burden on a therapist, a parent, a friend, or a spouse, a burden to be ever and always present and empathic lest we traumatize the other. Yet in my experience in each of these roles, I have not found that either negative affects or misattunements, in the majority of instances, resulted in experiences of trauma.

Differentiating the Repetition Compulsion

There seem to be at least two confusions or difficulties in this conceptualization. One has to do with using injury as a model for psychopathology, which, as I suggested above, may reflect psychiatry's close ties to medicine. I would argue that this model ties us too closely to spatial metaphors, as if a painful affective experience could actually leave some kind of physical injury that occurred at a particular moment or in a singular event. But in psychopathology it seems that what we are talking about most of the time is more like an underlying psychological vulnerability, which, I would argue, consists of an increased potential to feel overwhelmed by painful affects that one feels unable to control or to modulate either through one's own efforts or with the help of others. A shift from injury to vulnerability allows for a more variable range of possibilities. First of all, it highlights the intrapsychic experience of feeling overwhelmed with painful affects and feeling helpless to do anything about it. One can then begin to think of all the different kinds of conditions that would create, evoke, or reduce a vulnerability, conditions that could vary from person to person, and from time to time, or that could emerge from internal or external sources; that is, either the painful affects or the failure to cope with them can emerge from intrapsychic or interpersonal sources. Such a formulation also allows for variations in the degree of vulnerability and thus of psychic pain, so that under some conditions pain can be bearable and nontraumatic. And finally it shifts us away from a process of healing to a process of decreasing vulnerability through containment, tolerance, and an increase in mastery of painful affects. The goal, then, is not to rid ourselves of vulnerability but to reduce its parameters (its scope and intensity) to more manageable dynamics.

The second confusion has to do with using the term *trauma* so broadly that important distinctions between qualities of psychic pain and resources for enduring, tolerating, or mastering pain are obscured. Here I am referring to qualitative distinctions between affects, quantitative distinctions based on varying intensities of each affect, and a whole range of variables, both intrapsychic and interpersonal, that can be considered as constituting resources for managing painful affects. For, although all psychological defensive mechanisms are created by individuals to protect the psyche from feeling overwhelmed by painful affects that are imagined to be too painful and/or too uncontrollable to know about or to endure, nevertheless not all defensive strategies are the same in terms of their scope, their flexibility, their urgency, their ultimate goals, and their effectiveness. Indeed, we have several formulations suggesting hierarchies of defenses ranging from primitive to neurotic to adaptive. Thus it seems impossible to reconcile Russell's ubiquitous use of the term *trauma* with these important distinctions.

Later I shall try to demonstrate how important these distinctions can be clinically. I shall argue that there is a difference between the affects and the defensive organization and goals operating in what has been called the repetition compulsion, and the affects and defensive organization and goals most often involved in cases of trauma. But since the distinctions I am arguing for are based on certain assumptions about the nature of affects, their dynamics, and their function, it is necessary first to clarify the differences in my approach to and understanding of affect from those expressed by Russell and by other relational and interpersonal psychoanalytic writers.

In Russell's discussion of affects, he places the relationship at the center of his conceptualization. Thus affects are object seeking, the capacity to feel never develops in isolation, one needs a relationship to discover what one feels, and so forth. This is a conceptualization common to other interpersonalists and object relation perspectives. It seems to derive primarily from the therapeutic, clinical setting in which failures in adaptation predominate, and in which the process of bringing about a change in adaptive functioning requires the creation and use of a therapeutic relationship. I do not disagree with the central importance of the relationship in therapeutic work and in development, but even in these contexts, I am arguing that it is neither necessary nor particularly helpful to assume that affective experience can occur only within a relationship. Elsewhere, I have written more extensively about the theoretical limitations of this stance (Demos 1996). Here I would briefly suggest that it obscures the biological and psychological (intrapsychic) nature, functions, and dynamics of affects, of development, of psychopathology, and of the therapeutic process.

The most comprehensive and systematic theory of affect has come not out of psychoanalysis, but rather from the work of Silvan S. Tomkins, a philosopher turned psychologist. His theory of discrete affects has spawned a resurgence of interest and research in affects in a variety of fields. In psychology, Tomkins's specification of the importance of the face in affective experience led to the development of methodologies for coding facial expressions (see Ekman 1982, Ekman, Friesen, and Tomkins 1971, and Izard 1971, 1977), which has resulted in an extraordinary increase in research on infant affect. In psychiatry, there has been a gradual reexamination of the importance of affects (to name only two, see Basch 1976 and Nathanson 1992). And more recently Tomkins's work has been of use to literary scholars (Sedgewick and Frank 1995).

In volume 1 of his four-volume work entitled *Affect, Imagery, Consciousness* (*A.I.C.*), Tomkins wrote about the evolution of affects and suggested that "natural selection has operated on man to heighten three distinct classes of affect—affect for the preservation of life, affect for people and affect for novelty" (1962, p. 27). This is a profound departure from Freud's notion that all of human functioning derives from aggression or libido, and from a relational stance that insists that all affects are object seeking. Tomkins is unique in appreciating both the importance and the distinct motivational underpinnings of the human capacity to respond to novelty, thereby providing a more flexible and comprehensive understanding of human functioning. Thus, for example, the human capacity to become deeply engaged in exploring the inanimate world does not have to be understood as a derivative of libido or of object relations. It can operate independently and indeed may at times come in conflict with these other needs: "There could be no guarantee that selection for social responsiveness might not conflict with selection for self-preservative responsiveness and with selection for curiosity and responsiveness to novelty and thus complicate the problem of the integration of these characteristics" (Tomkins 1962, p. 27).

Staying with this biological perspective for the moment, I would like to focus on the capacity to feel affect. Tomkins argues that as products of a long evolutionary history, human beings are born with the capacity to experience the full range of basic affects, which have been described as enjoyment, interest, distress, anger, fear, startle, disgust, and shame. Although there are only meager data on neonatal facial, vocal, and autonomic behaviors, I have argued elsewhere (Demos 1988, 1992) that these data are in agreement with Tomkins's formulation. He defines these experiences as the result of affect programs, which are correlated sets of responses including facial expressions, vocalizations, respiratory patterns, autonomic responses (heart rate, skin temperature, viscera), and skeletal responses. These affect programs function as general and abstract amplifiers of stimuli impinging on the organism and create, through facial, vocal, and autonomic responses, an analogue that is experienced as inherently rewarding or inherently punishing. Tomkins postulates that there are both innate and learned activators of affect, and that each discrete affect is activated by a particular pattern of stimulation, such as increases and decreases in rates of stimulation densities and differing levels of non-optimal stimulation. When internal or external sources of neural firing suddenly increase, the organism will startle, become afraid, or become interested depending on the suddenness of the rate of the increase. When sources of neural firing reach and maintain a high non-optimal level of stimulation, the organism will experience distress or anger, depending on the level of stimulation. And when the sources of neural firing suddenly decrease, the organism will laugh or smile with enjoyment depending on the suddenness of the decrease. Shame is activated when positive affect (e.g., interest–excitement) is interrupted and attenuated without being completely reduced.

Tomkins distinguishes between the affect program per se and affect-related information that may include the perceived trigger of an affect; the response to an affect, including memories, plans, fantasies, perceptions; and motor responses that may or may not be co-assembled with an affect at any given moment. He refers to these co-assemblies as affect complexes or as ideo–affect organizations. Ideo–affect is an abbreviation for ideation–perception–memory–action–affect, which refers to the involvement of all of the critical subsystems that together constitute a human being, and that are all operational in the newborn infant. Ideo–affect complexes are constructed over time as the infant experiences emotions and gradually connects these experiences to a variety of antecedents and to a variety of outcomes or consequences, a process that enables the infant to organize and learn to manage affective experiences.

The newborn infant, then, has the capacity to experience affect but does not yet have past experience to draw on. Thus the crying neonate knows neither why she is crying nor that there is anything that can be done about it. The cry in this initial experience represents an innate affective response to a continuous level of non-optimal stimulation such as hunger or fatigue, which, in conjunction with a correlated set of facial-muscle, blood-flow, visceral, respiratory, and skeletal responses, will amplify the original stimulus and produce an inherently painful experience of distress for the infant. As Tomkins has said, "affect either makes good things better or bad things worse" (1978, p. 203). In contrast to Freud's (1895) idea that crying (affect) represents a discharge of drive tension, Tomkins argues that crying (distress) amplifies the tension and makes it feel worse. The adaptive evolutionary function of such an amplifying mechanism is to make the organism care about what is happening (what is changing or staying the same at non-optimal levels) and to motivate the organism to organize a response. For Tomkins, affects are the primary motivators.

These patterned facial, vocal, autonomic, and motor affect programs are not learned: every neonate knows how to cry in distress or in anger. Nor do they operate in a reflex-like manner; they are exquisitely responsive to subtle changes in the internal or external environment. Nor do they require the presence of a caregiver for the infant to know that they are occurring or that they are painful. Affect is *always* an intrapsychic experience combining urgency, abstractness, and generality (e.g., too much, too fast, just right) with a qualitative coloring of pain or pleasure. It may or may not also be an interpersonal experience. The fact that affective experiences occur most frequently in relationship to others should not obscure the fact that they can and do occur independently of others. For example, if a hungry infant is left alone and allowed to cry for an extended period of time, as occurred in institutions several decades ago and may still occur in some homes, innate affect dynamics will cause the infant to cycle up into higher and higher densities of distress and anger (and possibly fear, depending on the rate of increase) and eventually to fall asleep from exhaustion. But this is such an extremely painful experience that the infant will eventually learn to prevent its recurrence by learning not to cry. Such an infant stops crying not because a caregiver actively discouraged it, but because there was no caregiver and no relationship to a caregiver to help the infant manage such overwhelming intrapsychic experiences. The possibility of this kind of intrapsychic affect experience and intrapsychic efforts to manage it does not seem to be easily formulated or acknowledged within a relational or interpersonal perspective.

If the caregiver is not necessary for the infant to experience an affect or to know that it is painful or pleasurable, or even to learn to avoid it, then what is the role of the caregiver with regard to affect? There are many things an infant must learn in order to organize these affective experiences, most of which can be learned only from other human beings. This learning begins very early in the context of the infant–caregiver dyad and continues throughout life. It includes cultural, familial, and personal meanings and expressive forms, such as what and how much can be expressed to whom, when, in what form, and to what end, what can be talked about, or never mentioned, or never named, or never even thought (Demos 1993). In early infancy, however, the main role for the caregiver is in managing and modulating the intensity of negative affects.

Initially infants have only a very limited repertoire of responses for managing experiences of distress, anger, fear, or startle, and these work best at relatively low levels of intensity. But beyond these low levels of distress or fussiness, infants do not possess the instrumental capacities, the experience, or the knowledge to help themselves. They need a responsive caregiver to help them modulate and manage more intense negative affects and to protect them from overwhelming escalations of negative affects. But since negative affects are an inescapable part of living, and since they have evolved as amplifiers, making things feel worse in order to motivate us by making us care about what is happening, then the developmental task, and I would argue the therapeutic task, is to learn to be able to tolerate and endure our affects so as to use the information contained in them and to organize an adaptive response. I am suggesting that there is an optimal density (intensity times duration) of negative affect that is neither too little, thereby preventing the infant/child/patient from exercising and developing his or her regulatory capacities, nor too much, thereby overwhelming the infant/child/patient and evoking defensive responses, but that ranges from moderate to moderately dense. This optimal level will vary from person to person, from moment to moment, from context to context, and is therefore difficult to specify. But it is nevertheless recognizable, because it is a level that will allow the infant/child/patient to remain in the situation, to continue to organize these experiences, and to try to do something about the situation.

The caregiver's dual role as protector and modulator is crucial for the infant/child. For if the caregiver succeeds in maintaining the infant's/child's experience of negative affects within optimal densities, the result will be a sense of trust within the infant/child, a trust in the reliability and manageability of one's inner experiences. The infant/child will have learned that the onset of negative affect does not signal the end of a task, or a dreaded escalation, but rather that the experience can be borne, that finding a resolution is possible, and that the painful quality of the experience will come to an end. The infant/child will also learn that the caregiver is reliable, that one can depend on help from other people, and that the world is trustworthy. Both kinds of learning will happen simultaneously, and both are important. But to learn that one's insides are reliable, manageable, and bearable will enable the infant/child to remain in distressing, or maddening, or frightening situations when alone and to develop a variety of adaptive solutions. It will also enable her to tolerate the distress, anger, and/or fear of others, and will enhance her capacities to probe and explore her own as well as others' inner experiences, without having to worry about being surprised, overwhelmed, or disorganized by intense negative affects, and therefore without having to defend against such experiences.

This, then, is the first area of difference between myself and Russell. Based on Tomkins's theory of affects, I am arguing for the need to include in our clinical formulations the possibility that affective experiences can arise outside of relationships, and the need to recognize that even within the relational context, when intrapsychic and interpersonal processes are intermingled and simultaneous, they nevertheless can be and often are quite distinguishable and separate.

The second area of difference between myself and Russell has to do with making qualitative distinctions between negative affects and the kinds of defensive strategies these distinct affects engender. I shall focus particularly on differentiating the defensive strategies involved in the repetition compulsion from those involved in trauma. Again I shall rely heavily on Tomkins's theory of discrete affects and shall briefly describe his script theory, which deals with defensive organizations. Tomkins argues that each of the basic affects has particular characteristics and functions, and that "some affects are better than others for human beings, and some are very lethal" (1995d, p. 395). For the purposes of this discussion I will focus on only the negative affects, namely shame, distress, disgust, anger, and fear. I have listed these in the order of the least toxic to the most toxic according to Tomkins's formulation.

Tomkins defines shame as an affect auxiliary, which is triggered by a temporary interruption of or any perceived impediment to the continuation of either excitement or enjoyment. Thus he views shame as an affluent emotion, since it arises only in the context of strong positive affects focused on the other or on some aspect of the world. Distress is activated by a continuing level of non-optimal neural stimulation that occurs across a wide variety of stimuli and accounts for the ubiquity of human suffering. Thus he sees distress as a fundamental human emotion and contrasts it to fear–anxiety, which he sees as an emergency affect.

> It seems very likely that the differentiation of distress from fear was required in part because the coexistence of superior cognitive powers of anticipation, with an affect as toxic as fear, could have destroyed man if this were the only affect expressing suffering. What was called

for was a less toxic, but still negative, affect which would motivate human beings to solve disagreeable problems without too great a physiological cost or too great a probability of running away from the many problems that confront the human being and which would permit anticipation of trouble at an optimal psychic and biological cost. Such, we think, is the human cry of distress. [1995a, p. 73][1]

Tomkins describes disgust as a drive-auxiliary response, as in vomiting out bad food that when eaten was thought to be good. When used metaphorically, disgust is a response of disenchantment to people and events, in which both "dis-" and "enchantment" are important elements. It has thus taken on a more general motivating function, so that humans react with disgust to others, to themselves, and to events as if these entities were bad food that once had been good. I believe that this affect has been greatly underappreciated in clinical work and writings, with the result that much of the toxicity attributed to shame is probably mistaken and would more accurately be identified as a manifestation of disgust, which when turned on the self can generate profound self-loathing.

Fear–terror and anger–rage are viewed by Tomkins as the most toxic affects. Fear is activated by a rapid rate of increase in stimulation; it is physiologically costly to the organism and is designed to function as an emergency affect in life-threatening situations. Anger is triggered by a higher level of non-optimal stimulation and is therefore more toxic than distress. Rage, as opposed to distress, does not lend itself to fine, long-term use.

---

1. See Tomkins 1963, which is volume 2 of *A.I.C.*, for a more detailed and rich discussion of shame and distress.

(See Tomkins 1991, which is volume 3 of *A.I.C.*, for an extraordinary and exhaustive discussion of fear and anger.)

According to Tomkins, these characteristic differences among the negative affects are systematically related to the kinds of strategies, which he calls scripts, that human beings create to manage them. He makes an important distinction between the amplification that is produced momentarily by the activation of an affect, with its correlated set of responses, and what he calls psychological magnification, which involves an active process of connecting two affect-laden scenes across time. Magnification increases both the affective power of each scene and their relatedness to each other. Thus

> in affect magnification, cognitive, motor, perceptual, and memorial processes are centrally involved, because magnification requires the formation of a script, which is time binding. Affect is momentary; in general, it is of short duration. That is inherent in the mechanism. Were we dependent upon that all of our life, we would be very impoverished human beings. But we are not impoverished. We are not impoverished because we can bring all of our resources to bear on the scenes we experience, co-assemble them, consider their relationships, and design strategies to deal with them in the future. This I have called a set of rules—compressed rules—and labeled them scripts. [1995b, p. 289]

Tomkins has written extensively on scripts, their formation, and different classes of scripts (see 1992 and 1995c). What follows is a very brief description of some of the general features of scripts and of their formation. They are sets of ordering rules for the interpretation, evaluation, prediction, production, or control of scenes. They are selective in terms of the number and types of scenes they order, they are incomplete, and they vary in their accuracy. Because of their selectivity, incompleteness, and inaccuracy, they are continually reordered and changing. Thus, initially, the scenes determine the script, and the criteria for inclusion can be quite selective. But over time, as the number of connected scenes increases, and/or as the urgency to manage the scenes increases, the script determines the scenes. Thus most scripts become more self-validating than self-fulfilling.

In Tomkins's formulation, a scene is the basic unit of analysis of psychological experience. It is a happening with a perceived beginning and an end, which includes at least one affect in a particular context, for example, place, action, and people. But the important point for script theory is that no single scene or set of scenes occurring at any moment in time, no matter how intense or painful, can have an enduring effect until the future happens and either further magnifies this experience or attenuates it. Tomkins argues further that the consequence of any experience is not singular but plural, with many effects that change in time. For example, how often will a person rehearse a set of bad scenes over time, and will this use of imagination in terms of the way the scenes are ordered or spaced, be experienced as magnifying or attenuating the painful affects? What other events will occur that will be perceived as similar? Magnification occurs, not by repetition, but by repetition with a difference: "Any scene which is sufficiently similar to evoke the same kind of affect is thereby made more similar, and increases the degree of connectedness of the whole family of scenes" (1995c, p. 326). A script is created to deal with the individual's rules for predicting, interpreting, responding to, and controlling a magnified set of scenes.

I have introduced Tomkins's script theory because it provides a comprehensive way to understand personality formation and organization. Script theory was conceptualized as a general personality theory. Its advantages over previous formulations were succinctly described by Brewster Smith (1995), an eminent personality psychologist, in his introduction to the edited volume of the selected writings of Silvan S. Tomkins:

> Script theory seems to me to provide the coherent framework for the dynamic (motivational) characterization of personality that the field badly needs. . . . [A]s a developmental conception regarding the conditional linkage of "scenes" and affects in a person's life, it affords an extremely flexible language for analyzing personality structure and processes. It is based on human universals—the affects and the scripting process—but readily accommodates cultural and individual specificity of scenes and sequences. It therefore immediately escapes the culture-boundedness and history-boundedness of all standard personality theories . . . and provides a language for the idiographic treatment of personal uniqueness. It is committed neither to unity nor to fragmentation in personality organization, neither to inner-directed nor to other-directed role-playing versions of personality. It is truly general in its applications and claims. . . . [S]cript theory flatly rejects the energy metaphors of drive theory. . . . [I]t is saved from dehumanizing ethical relativism by its linkage to Tomkins's polarity theory and his doctrines concerning the socialization of positive and negative affects. There are better and worse ways of being a person and Tomkins's theory can be articulate about them. [p. 10]

I would add that because it can encompass both adaptive and non-adaptive personality organizations, it is useful to clinicians and relevant to our discussion.

If we now return to the negative affects described earlier, we can explore how each of these affects, if sufficiently magnified in a life, will become scripted. Tomkins has argued that a class of scripts that he defined as risk, cost-benefit scripts fits rather well with the distinct characteristics of each of the basic affects. Briefly, these are described as follows. Affluent scripts deal with the positive affects of enjoyment and interest, which we have not focused on in this discussion. Damage-reparation scripts deal with scenes that are affluent but have suffered some damage, which could be repaired. Shame is the dominant affect in these scripts, since it is an auxiliary affect to enjoyment and interest, activated by an interruption of or perceived impediment to these affects. Thus damage-reparation scripts are relatively optimistic, involving strategies that perceive costs and risks as relatively low or tolerable for the benefits of reestablishing positive affect. Limitation-remediation scripts deal with scenes of permanent or enduring problems, such as death of a loved one, handicaps, chronic disease, or limitations in opportunity. These are serious problems that, however, can be confronted and improved or remedied in some way. Distress, which lends itself to long-term coping with stressful situations, is the dominant affect in these scripts. They make use of an optimizing strategy in which one accepts and endures the pain of distress (cost) and the risks of loss or trouble in order to optimize the possible benefits of positive engagement. Decontamination scripts deal with scenes that involve the dynamics of disgust. These are scenes that were once enchanting but have become contaminated or spoiled in some way. The experience is not one of a damage that can be repaired, or of a limitation or problem that can be remedied; it is rather an experience of impurity or contamination that must be expunged, purified, or decontaminated. Such scripts make use of a maximizing–minimizing strategy, seeking nothing less than purification in an attempt to minimize any possibility or risk of contamination, which is experienced as highly painful. As you can see, these scripts are moving from bad to worse. The final set of scripts are anti-toxic scripts that deal with scenes of intolerable pain, scenes that evoke intense terror and/or rage. These scenes must be avoided, eliminated, or escaped; thus psychic energy is devoted entirely to prevention. In these strategies risk is maximized because the cost is intolerable, and benefit is defined only as the absence of risk or of intolerable pain. Thus hypervigilance and avoidance dominate.

These scripts can co-exist with each other in a personality, although the more urgent and painful the affect, the more likely it is to dominate. Thus decontamination scripts powered by disgust and anti-toxic scripts powered by terror and/or rage tend to monopolize psychic energy and crowd out other scripting possibilities.

I have presented this brief description of Tomkins's script theory and of these negative-affect scripts in order to set the stage for the discussion of the distinction between the repetition compulsion and its dynamics and the dynamics involved in trauma. As you can now perhaps anticipate, I would like to suggest that Tomkins's formulation of decontamination scripts offers a way to understand what is occurring dynamically in the repetition compulsion, and that his definition of anti-toxic scripts may help us understand the effects of trauma on the psyche.

There has been a great deal of discussion in the psychoanalytic literature about what Freud, and others since Freud, have meant by repetition and the repetition compulsion. Recently, Wilson and Malatesta (1989) have provided an interesting review and excellent discussion of these issues. They describe the effort to distinguish a broad definition, namely, the general phenomena of repetition that occur in the transference, in all of our relationships, as well as in all kinds of learning throughout our lives (e.g., as in practicing), from the more limited or specific definition of the phenomena motivating a compulsion to repeat. Russell also feels this distinction is important and includes biological processes in his general formulation of repetition. Tomkins too makes a distinction between what he calls duplication, which he describes as a general biological process inherent in all living organisms, and repetition, which he defines in terms of psychological perceptual experience. He argues that simple repetition leads to boredom and to sensory habituation. What captures the psyche and evokes interest is repetition with a difference. The repetition compulsion, then, must have this characteristic of repetition with a difference, whatever else may be involved in generating the compulsion.

Beyond this general distinction between a broad definition of repetition and the more circumscribed definition of the repetition compulsion, which it seems everyone would accept, Wilson and Malatesta go on to focus on what is being repeated in a repetition compulsion. They review Freud's reasoning in *Beyond the Pleasure Principle* (1920), to which Russell also makes reference. In this article Freud struggled to reconcile his discovery that dreams contain wishes with his observation that some dreams, namely nightmares, produce negative affects; thus the person seems to be wishing for an experience of painful affects, and in flashbacks for a repetition of a painful experience. Was this wish in the service of mastery of these painful experiences? Freud's solution to what he saw as masochism was to evoke the death instinct. Wilson and Malatesta argue that this solution was so unsatisfactory that it led to an avoidance of this topic for several decades. They suggest that now (in 1989), given the increases in our knowledge of infancy and advances in psychoanalytic theory, we are in a position to revisit this issue of the repetition compulsion. They propose that there are primal, preconscious, non-symbolic affective interactive patterns, acquired early in life, that remain outside of our awareness, beyond subjectivity, which constitute the contents of the repetition compulsion. They contrast these patterns with patterns that involve symbolic fantasies and wishes that occur after the advent of language and that are therefore more amenable to consciousness and to therapeutic intervention. These they would call transference, a more general form of repetition.

I find their solution to the problem as unsatisfactory as Freud's earlier resort to the death instinct. There are several difficulties. First of all, since we all possess these early, presymbolic patterns, it would seem that we all therefore must be struggling with some form of the repetition compulsion. Yet, in my clinical experience, this is clearly not the case. To the contrary, this kind of pathology is particularly difficult to treat and is more likely to result in a negative therapeutic response than other kinds of problems. Secondly, Wilson and Malatesta are assuming that presymbolic experience is somehow preconscious when it happens and remains outside of our awareness once we attain symbolic capacities. I would argue that there is no evidence to support such a general claim. Infants are conscious and aware as they experience their lives, and they organize their experiences using whatever schemes they can create at the time. And—recall Tomkins's useful distinction between amplification and magnification—they will continue to reorganize their experience as they perceive connections between the present and the recent past. Because this process of reorganization is continuous, as they become capable of symbolic mental activity these early experiences will continue to become part of new organizations and will become symbolized in one form or another. Clearly, not everything will be put into language, but that is also true of experiences we have throughout our lives; it is not unique to our earliest experiences. Language is a tremendous gain in all kinds of ways, but it is always an imperfect tool for expressing the totality of our experiences (Stern 1985). Thirdly, even if Wilson and Malatesta had limited their claim (which they didn't) to the kind of aberrant early experiences described by Bion (1967) as beta elements, or by Mitrani (1995) as unmentalized experiences that are thought to remain unsymbolized, this would still be an unsatisfactory solution. Recall that Freud's criterion for the repetition compulsion involved experiences that had achieved symbolic representation in the form of images in dreams and flashbacks.

But the most serious difficulty with their solution is that it fails to account for the compulsion. In their formulation, the motivation for repetition is not specified; it is neither a wish to master painful affect, nor a masochistic dance with the death instinct, but rather a variety of wishes embedded in early interactional patterns. These patterns are subtle and difficult to become aware of and are therefore difficult to intervene with in therapy or to change. But the nature and even the affective valence of these early motivations are left unspecified. So although they provide some push for gratification, the compulsion for repeating seems to occur mainly because we cannot get hold of them. They are seen as primal and beyond subjectivity. Thus the whole paradox of repeating painful and what appear to be self-defeating behaviors does not take center stage in this formulation.

Russell emphasizes the painful affects involved in the repetition compulsion and in the treatment of such patients. He seems to assume that these painful states are sought in an effort to master them. Others have argued that when negative therapeutic reactions occur, one is dealing with a strong attachment to early painful experiences with caregivers and with a refusal to give up this attachment. In both of these two latter formulations there is an emphasis on seeking pain or negative affect, and the sense that the patients are unable to or refuse to grieve the loss of something they either never had or that they cannot now find. In my experience, this refusal to grieve is only half the story. I would argue that in the repetition compulsion, the repetition of painful affects is *not* the goal. It is instead the unanticipated consequence of a failed strategy. Patients are not seeking painful affects; they are trying neither to hold onto the destructiveness of the caregiver nor to master painful affects. They are seeking something else entirely, and they seek it repeatedly. But their strategy is deeply flawed and thus they fail repeatedly, thereby experiencing painful affect. What is this flawed strategy that is being compulsively repeated? We need to return to Tomkins's decontamination script.

A decontamination script adopts a maximizing–minimizing strategy that seeks nothing less than purification, perfection, and decontamination in an attempt to minimize the risk of feeling the self-disgust of contamination that contains within it a deep sense of unacceptable badness, an inherent rottenness that is believed to be sickening to behold. As a therapist, one becomes aware of how the internal world of these patients has become dynamically polarized into two idealized opposites, namely an imagined paradise that never really existed in the past but that they continually seek, even though it is not actually attainable in the present, and a hell that is imagined to be more disgusting than could ever have been true in the past and that they try desperately not to revisit, even though it is not as unacceptable as they imagine it to be in the present. The vast middle realm of possibilities seems outside of their experience.

People who have needed to create this script in order to manage a whole family of earlier painful and deeply ambivalent scenes are caught in a repeating cycle of becoming enchanted or seduced by a love possibility and/or a work opportunity that evokes in them some version of the fantasy "now all my problems will be solved," with the emphasis on *all*. There is an unrealistic, grandiose, naive belief in the possibility of a life without pain, the end of all suffering. With each new possibility, they may be able to deny or ignore any sign of trouble for quite a while. But, since trouble is an ordinary part of life, their strategy is doomed to fail. Sooner or later, inevitably, the enchantment is spoiled by an undeniable flaw in the other or an unavoidable difficulty or problem at work. When such a realization comes, it produces a massive, rapid plunge into the depths of self-doubt, despair, disgust, and contamination. There are many versions of this rapid downward plunge, which often involve projecting blame all over the place. But, ultimately, these patients believe deep down that their inherent rottenness is to blame for whatever went wrong, which is an equally grandiose fantasy. It is the unbearableness of this conviction that compels the person to seek an escape in the fantasy of purification and leads them into the next round of seduction.

There is remarkably little learning from one enchantment–disenchantment cycle to the next. Each time feels entirely new, different from the past and very promising. Tomkins (1995c) has described this dynamic cycle and polarity as a combination of greed and cowardice. The greed involves the grandiose fantasy of perfection, a belief that one could actually escape suffering, and the loading of each new situation with such unrealistic expectations. The cowardice comes with imagining that it would be impossible to ever face one's failings, one's incapacities, one's vengeful fantasies, which have also been exaggerated into grandiose proportions. Herein lies the refusal to grieve for the ordinary limitations or losses in life. But both ends of this polarity must be present and exaggerated in order for repetition to become compulsive.

The seduction must always occur first, not only in the present, but in the past as well. Remember that disgust is evoked when one has taken something in that was believed to be good, even wonderful, and then turns rotten, but now that rottenness is inside oneself and must be expunged. What kind of early experiences lead to such a script? In my experience both as a therapist and as a supervisor, these patients grew up with parents who seem to have been struggling with this same deeply ambivalent, polarized split within themselves. But as parents they attempt to hoard all the goodness and may present themselves as wonderful, loving, perfect parents, projecting badness outward, onto the world, and/or onto the child. Again, there are many ways in which this can happen, but the essential ingredients seem to involve (1) a seductive, even charismatic quality in the parent, who conveys his or her investment in the child with fervor, with ideological conviction, or with intimidating and intrusive power, so that either the child's imagination is seized with the wish to please, to join, to be close to this idealized other, or the child feels compelled out of weakness to join, and harbors secret revenge fantasies of counteractive power. This must be combined with (2) the parent's intolerance of any sign in the child of "badness": not complying with the parent's needs, not validating the parent's goodness, or simply irritating the parent, so that when the child fails, as the child will inevitably do, the parent both exaggerates the seriousness of the failure and conveys the unacceptability and intolerance of such qualities, behaviors, and/or feelings. Thus these are initially good scenes that have turned very bad, and they are extremely painful for the child to experience, not only because disgust is a powerfully negative feeling and may involve the child's awareness of his/her own complicity in what transpires, but also because these children are often left alone to try to cope with their parent's devastating judgment and rejection of them, leaving them feeling helpless and devalued. As small children, they cannot step back and accurately assess the appropriateness either of their behavior or of their parent's reactions. And the more alone, helpless, and devalued these children feel, the less they can imagine themselves as the source of anything good, and the more powerful and desirable their parents seem, as the parents come to represent the promise of everything good. Therefore, over time, the child comes to believe that this exaggerated badness, which is both projected onto them by the parent and confirms the child's own inner experience of weakness and vengefulness, is a valid assessment of their true nature. Because of this congruence between the child's secret thoughts and wishes and the parents' judgment, the child then believes that he/she is the source of all badness, which feels unbearable, and so the decontamination fantasy takes hold and this script is created. Thus a child's clinging to an abusive parent, or a wife's staying with an abusive husband, is not motivated by a wish for punishment but occurs because often these same abusive others are also the source of the child's or the wife's most rewarding positive scenes and the potential source of a fantasied confession and redemption.

TRAUMA, REPETITION, AND AFFECT REGULATION

In the treatment of this powerful, repetitive, doomed-to-fail strategy, which I believe is what is meant by the repetition compulsion, the transference will alternate between idealizing the therapist, for example expecting the therapist to provide all the necessary knowledge and power to bring about a cure, and experiencing the therapist as critical, controlling, and intrusive. It is necessary to work on recognizing, identifying, and putting into words both the unrealistic, grandiose expectations and fantasies of perfection and the exaggerated, grandiose sense of badness, and to provide a framework to explore this polarized internal world. Once patients begin to identify the underlying similarity of the wish in their grandiose fantasies, and begin to recognize the repetitions, they can begin to imagine, at least intellectually, a more realistic, normalized, humanized world. But the emotional work, and the key to this process, involves helping them to give voice to and to tolerate their imagined badness. This phase of therapy is, I believe, what Russell described so well with his notion of a paradox, namely creating safety that then invites painful affects that may disrupt the treatment. For patients will struggle valiantly not to sit with these feelings or to acknowledge how truly rotten they feel themselves to be. They may try to project this badness onto the therapist, they may harbor the hope for some miraculous escape from this process, they may cut themselves or engage in bingeing and purging trying to rid themselves of the badness and of the therapy process. The therapist must be able to contain all of this disgust, rage, hatred, longing, and fear, so as to enable patients gradually to own both their susceptibility to seduction and the longings motivating it, and to tolerate their dreaded badness, which includes their fantasies of revenge and retroactive justice.

Differentiating the Repetition Compulsion

Once they can begin to find the courage to accept what they imagine to be the worst parts of themselves, the compulsion to seek purification in an endless cycle of enchantment and disenchantment begins to decrease markedly. They then, gradually, become better and better at recognizing within themselves all the ways in which they are tempted to idealize or to become seduced again, and, when disappointed, all the ways they are seized by a wish for vengeance. The therapy begins to enter into a phase in which the grieving process is prominent. They grieve the loss of fantasies of confessions and justice that can never come true, of the kind of childhood they never had and that can never be redone, of years of abandoning themselves to the wishes of others, and the loss of a more grandiose world. They begin to feel more real in the sessions, more grounded in reality. Obviously these phases of therapy are not as clean cut as I have made them sound. There is backsliding; there continue to be cycles. But there is nevertheless a perceptible gradual change, so that the seductions are not so compelling or long lasting, the plunges into self-loathing are not so deep and intractable, and there is a gradual entering into that vast middle realm of experience, where every event is no longer loaded with grandiose fantasies.

I would like to shift the discussion now to trauma, which, in my experience, seems to create a very different kind of dynamic organization, one that fits with Tomkins's definition of an antitoxic script. In this script, the goal is not to try to live out a fantasy of purification or perfection, but rather to defend the psyche from any possible situations, relationships, or thoughts that could lead to terror or rage. These affects are toxic and intolerable; thus the risk of encountering them is maximized because the cost of experiencing them is too high. The only benefit that can be imagined is an absence of the possibility of this threat of trouble.

Often this relief from threat can be achieved only when one is alone.

In contrast to Russell's more ubiquitous use of the term *trauma*, it seems important to preserve the use of that word to describe such toxic scenes. These are scenes in which terror and/or rage are evoked and from which there is no escape. Such scenes can involve abusive others (e.g., beatings, sexual molestation), or they can involve destructive powers unleashed by nature (e.g., floods, storms), or by man (e.g., war, bombings). They can happen at any time in a life. What seems to be crucial is that (1) there is no escape from these toxic affects, and (2) these toxic scenes are extended over time. The experience of being unable to escape these toxic affects is an important aspect of what sets this script apart from a decontamination script and the compulsion to repeat. The compulsion is an enactment of the fantasy that one can escape disgust and self-loathing, one can find purification and perfection. By contrast, in an anti-toxic script, there is no imaginable escape possible except death, so the goal is to prevent any recurrence of these affects. The extension over time is necessary for magnification of the original experience to occur. If the original trauma is responded to with successful treatment or help in coping with its effects, an anti-toxic script will not develop. The toxic experience must be magnified in order for the anti-toxic script to develop. This magnification, which takes place over time, can occur in several ways. The scenes can actually recur, as in war or in repeated parental abuse, so that the toxicity in the original scene is magnified both by the actual repetition of these scenes and by the anticipation in imagination of their recurrence, which magnifies the dread and the helplessness, thereby increasing the toxicity of the whole experience. Magnification can also occur because future events that are not themselves toxic may trigger flashbacks in which the original scenes and their toxic affects are relived.

Because these affects feel both intolerable and inescapable, the psyche tries to marshal all of its resources to prevent their recurrence, and this effort results in the formation of an anti-toxic script. This will involve the creation of massive defensive barriers, which almost always includes a highly developed hypervigilance that can become so automatic that such people cease to be aware of all the ways they have developed to avoid and to protect. They cannot afford to be caught unaware or to be surprised; thus control becomes primary and often involves a rigid control of the contents of consciousness, of thoughts, and of feelings, a shutting off of the mind, an inability to give in to sleep, and the like. People with anti-toxic scripts often develop passable social skills. But if their traumatic scenes involved abusive others, they can never allow themselves to get too close to anyone. The unpredictability of spontaneous human exchanges feels too dangerous. They cannot trust that these exchanges could be benign. Such people may become aware of a deep sense of isolation and loneliness, but this awareness may not feel painful enough for them to seek therapeutic help. If their anti-toxic script works and successfully protects them from intrusions of toxic affects, and they have not had to use alcohol, drugs, an eating disorder, or other health-threatening behaviors to help control their demons, or if they have not gotten into trouble using such tactics, then they may be able to live emotionally constricted but safe lives, without therapeutic help. But they remain walking time bombs.

Usually, what brings people with an anti-toxic script into treatment is a breakdown in the effectiveness of the script. Either events of life have overwhelmed them, for example the death of a parent or the loss of a job, or some situation or event has led to an unanticipated breakthrough of toxic affect, or they have miscalculated the capacity of their body to function with long-term use of alcohol or purging. They may be hospitalized because of an unsuccessful suicide attempt or a physical collapse. Occasionally a first hospitalization will lead to therapy, but more often they are treated only for their physical symptoms. They may go on for years, with occasional breakdowns in functioning but without any effort on their part or on the part of their caregivers to explore the underlying dynamics of their behavior or their crises. When they do come into treatment, it is because they realize they can no longer successfully control what is happening to them or protect themselves from horrible intrusions into consciousness of terror and/or rage. They can no longer feel safe *anywhere*, even when alone. But once in therapy, they initially only want help in reconstructing the defensive wall.

In order for patients with an anti-toxic script to get past the enormity of the risk they feel in taking down the defensive wall, they have to imagine that there is something else in life that they desire more than they desire safety. This something else that begins to evoke more powerful desires often involves a deep longing for intimacy with another human being. It can arise because the person has become a parent and feels a compelling need to relate to his or her child, or because some real relationship seems worth the effort, or because they have reached a point where a continued life of loneliness is no longer acceptable. But this commitment is shaky, because in addition to wanting more than safety, they have to believe that they have the courage, strength, and support to live through the process of facing what is behind the defensive wall. The possibility of change can feel very remote in the heat of the therapeutic work. It is dangerous and

Differentiating the Repetition Compulsion

difficult work, because these affects feel lethal and can lead to suicide or homicidal rage. The intolerable scenes the patient must try to detoxify are truly horrifying and may feel as traumatizing to the therapist as they do to the patient. Recent writings on trauma suggest the need for therapists to find and use supportive colleagues to help them bear the stress of this work (Pearlman and Saakvitne 1995, Wilson and Lindy 1994). The transferences in this kind of work are fluid and can shift rapidly. The therapist can suddenly become a terrifying and dangerous object for the patient, when the latter in is the throes of a terrifying memory that can feel very real and very present. Because these scenes were so overwhelming when they occurred initially, and because they have never been worked through and have continued to magnify in their toxicity, they can engulf the patient's psyche in the present with their realism. This is not a compulsion to repeat; it is an intrusion of unmetabolized toxic affect due to a breakdown or a relaxation of defenses. The therapist must remain steady and work to hold the patient in the here-and-now alliance as much as is possible in the face of these overwhelming, unmetabolized horrors.

The main point for this discussion is to stress how much more toxic and lethal these affects feel, and how much more rigid and desperate the defenses need to be in an anti-toxic script, where the only goal is safety from and prevention of the recurrence of these affects because there is no escape. In contrast, with a decontamination script that can be manifested in the compulsion to repeat, the person is dealing with disgust and the self-loathing it engenders, which, although painful, can be experienced, and is repeatedly experienced, precisely because the person imagines it can be escaped. Thus the defenses do not have to be so rigid. In the former case we see hypervigilance, massive inhibition of thought and affect, dissociation, numbing, insomnia, generalized anxiety, multiple substance abuse, and eating disorders, while in the latter case we see primarily projection, idealization, grandiosity, splitting, intellectualization, and some denial.

Both of these scripts can lead to loneliness and isolation. People in the grips of a decontamination script may stay hidden in relationships, fearing rejection if the other knew about their inherent badness or defectiveness. But such a person also believes he or she can attain purification or find perfection, and so is much more likely to take the necessary risks to achieve this goal. An anti-toxic strategy can also lead to hiding in relationships, particularly if the traumas have occurred at the hands of abusive others, but the avoidance of intimacy in this script is far more pervasive and extreme. It may involve dissociating at moments of potential closeness, because the consequences of a breakthrough of terror and/or rage are too toxic to risk. The ultimate solution in an anti-toxic script, if it stops working and can no longer protect the person from toxic affects, is death, either through murder of the threatening other or through suicide.

It is not uncommon for people who have developed an anti-toxic script also to have developed a decontamination script, so that even if they reach a point where they can relax their vigilance enough to engage in a relationship, they may feel too disgusting and bad because of their abusive history or their vengefulness to imagine that anyone could accept them or find them desirable. With therapeutic help, a person can move from an anti-toxic script to any of the other scripts described earlier, depending on what affective character issues existed before the traumatic events and their magnification occurred, although, as stated above, they often move to a decontamination script first. So too, people with a decontamination script can move to any other script, depending on other character issues, but most often they move first to a limitation-remediation script in which the capacity for grief and the letting go of old grievances are present.

CONCLUSION

I began my response to Russell with an appreciation of his description of working with patients in the heat of intense transference repetitions, and joined him in placing affects and affect dynamics at the center of pathology and treatment. I then went on to take issue with his more general statements about affects, the role of the relationship, trauma, and the repetition compulsion. In order to do that I needed to present a brief account of Tomkins's theory of discrete affects and of scripts. This enabled me to make a distinction between the biological function of affects that allows for the experience of affect to occur independently of relationships, and the process of organizing and modulating affective experiences that requires a relationship with other human beings. It also enabled me to describe the different qualities of negative affects and to relate these qualities systematically to the particular defensive organizations that Tomkins calls scripts. And finally, after a brief review of definitions of the repetition compulsion, including Russell's, I related the repetition compulsion to Tomkins's decontamination script and traumatic experiences to Tomkins's anti-toxic script.

My goal was to provide through Tomkins's theory a more differentiated and articulated classification of affects and their related defensive strategies than I felt was present in Russell's formulation of psychopathology and treatment, in which the term *trauma* was used ubiquitously. If affects play a central role in our work as clinicians, as both Russell and I would agree, then it is incumbent upon us to utilize the most systematic and articulate theory of affects available. I would argue that Tomkins's theory represents the state of the art at this time. It provides a more differentiated and articulated classification of affects. It distinguishes between the momentary amplification of affect and the time-binding process of magnification, in which one affect-laden scene from the past is connected to another affect-laden scene in the present in an ongoing effort to order, reorder, and manage affective experiences, until families of scenes come together to form a script, a set of organized rules. It offers a taxonomy of scripts that captures and encompasses both general and idiosyncratic features of lived experience. Building on all of the clinical insights from the past, I believe that, with Tomkins's comprehensive and systematic theory of affects and of scripts and their formation, we are now able to be much more precise and systematic in our thinking and in our approach to our patients, who continually challenge us with their suffering.

REFERENCES

Basch, M. F. (1976). The concept of affect: a re-examination. *Journal of the American Psychoanalytic Association* 24:759–777.

Bion, W. R. (1967). *Second Thoughts: Selected Papers on Psycho-analysis*. London: Heinemann.

Demos, E. V. (1988). Affect and the development of the self: a new frontier. In *Frontiers in Self Psychology: Progress in Self Psychology*, vol. 3, ed. A. Goldberg, pp. 27–35. Hillsdale, NJ: Analytic Press.

——— (1992). Silvan Tomkins's theory of emotion. In *Reinterpreting the Legacy of William James*, ed. M. E. Donnelly, pp. 211–219. Washington, DC: American Psychological Association.

——— (1993). Developmental foundations for the capacity for self-analysis: parallels in the roles of caregiver and analyst. In *Self-*

Analysis: Critical Inquiries, Personal Visions, ed. J. Barron, pp. 27–55. Hillsdale, NJ: Analytic Press.
——— (1995). *Exploring Affect: The Selected Writings of Silvan S. Tomkins.* New York: Cambridge University Press.
——— (1996). Expanding the interpersonal perspective. *Contemporary Psychoanalysis* 32(4):649–663.
Ekman, P. (1982). *Emotion in the Human Face: Guidelines for Research and an Integration of Findings*, 2nd. ed. New York: Cambridge University Press.
Ekman, P., Friesen, W. V., and Tomkins, S. (1971). Facial affect scoring technique: a first validity study. *Semiotica* 1:37–53.
Freud, S. (1895). Project for a scientific psychology. *Standard Edition* 1:283–387.
——— (1920). Beyond the pleasure principle. *Standard Edition* 18:8–68.
Izard, C. (1971). *The Face of Emotion.* New York: Appleton–Century Crofts.
——— (1977). *Human Emotions.* New York: Plenum.
Mitrani, J. L. (1995). Toward an understanding of unmentalized experience. *Psychoanalytic Quarterly* 64(1):68–112.
Nathanson, D. L. (1992). *Shame and Pride: Affect, Sex and the Birth of the Self.* New York: Norton.
Pearlman, L. A., and Saakvitne, K. W. (1995). *Trauma and the Therapist: Countertransference and Vicarious Traumatization in Psychotherapy with Incest Survivors.* New York: Norton.
Sedgewick, E. K., and Frank, A., eds. (1995). *Shame and Its Sisters: A Silvan Tomkins Reader.* Durham, NC: Duke University Press.
Smith, B. (1995). Introduction. In *Exploring Affect: The Selected Writings of Silvan S. Tomkins*, ed. E. V. Demos, pp. 1–12. New York: Cambridge University Press.
Stern, D. N. (1985). *The Interpersonal World of the Infant.* New York: Basic Books.
Tomkins, S. (1962). *Affect, Imagery, Consciousness, vol. 1. The Positive Affects.* New York: Springer.

——— (1963). *Affect, Imagery, Consciousness, vol. 2. The Negative Affects.* New York: Springer.

——— (1978). Script theory: differential magnification of affects. In *Nebraska Symposium on Motivation*, eds. H. E. Howe, Jr. and R. A. Dunstbier, pp. 201–236. Lincoln: University of Nebraska Press.

——— (1991). *Affect, Imagery, Consciousness, vol. 3. The Negative Affects Anger and Fear.* New York: Springer.

——— (1992). *Affect, Imagery, Consciousness, vol. 4. Cognition: Duplication and Transformation of Information.* New York: Springer.

——— (1995a). Role of the specific affects. In *Exploring Affect: The Selected Writings of Silvan S. Tomkins*, ed. E. V. Demos, pp. 68–85. New York: Cambridge University Press.

——— (1995b). Inverse archeology: facial affect and the interfaces of scripts within and between persons. In *Exploring Affect: The Selected Writings of Silvan S. Tomkins*, ed. E. V. Demos, pp. 284–290. New York: Cambridge University Press.

——— (1995c). Script theory. In *Exploring Affect: The Selected Writings of Silvan S. Tomkins*, ed. E. V. Demos, pp. 312–388. New York: Cambridge University Press.

——— (1995d). Revisions in script theory. In *Exploring Affect: The Selected Writings of Silvan S. Tomkins*, ed. E. V. Demos, pp. 389–396. New York: Cambridge University Press.

Wilson, A., and Malatesta, C. (1989). Affect and the compulsion to repeat: Freud's repetition compulsion revisited. *Psychoanalysis and Contemporary Thought* 12(2):265–312.

Wilson, J. P. and Lindy, J. D., eds. (1994). *Countertransference in the Treatment of P. T. S. D.* New York: Guilford.

SIX

PARADOX AND THE COGNITIVE FUNCTION OF AFFECT: A DISCUSSION OF RUSSELL'S PAPERS

George G. Fishman, M.D.

> Someday you be walking down the road and you hear something or see something going on. So clear. And you think it's you thinking it up. A thought picture. But no. It's when you bump into a rememory that belongs to somebody else.
> —TONI MORRISON, *Beloved*

INTRODUCTION

The publication of these two remarkable papers by Paul Russell will, I hope, be the beginning of a wide circulation of his work and integration of his ideas into the lively discourse of contemporary psychoanalysis. Paul's thinking resonates closely with the major currents in our literature: relational theory, intersubjectivity, trauma, affect, emergence, dynamic systems, connectionism, language philosophy. Although I will allude to the correspondence between Paul's ideas and those of others, my discussion will focus on the task that for me has highest priority: the elucidation of Paul's ideas in a way that is as close to their own terms as is possible. Paul was intrigued by Sylvan Tomkins's (1962) writings on affect. Tomkins believed that affects were acquired in evolution in order to interpret raw perception. In his view, affects provided analogic amplification of sensory data in order to give them a "point" or meaning. Amplification is the operative word. I want to exercise the same function with respect to the wealth Paul has offered us in these two texts. In a similar way, I will try to amplify key themes in the texts, so as to underline, clarify, and unpack their meanings. The anecdotes and examples I will offer all happened in the sense that Paul understood history: "There is . . . no such thing as a final, objective historical account. However, once one grants this, one discovers an internal logic to the successive unfolding of affective awareness that allows one to say, with as much certainty as is possible anywhere, that this or that must have been real. Here again, one discovers the internal logic, the necessary mathematics, of affective competency" (this volume, p. 38).

CONTAINMENT

Paul Russell did what he wrote. He was quintessential containment. I know because I, like many others who knew him as teacher, therapist, and friend, frequently presented him with my oil spills. I found out how he absorbed things in the first week of our meeting at the end of my residency in 1973. He was known on the residency grapevine as a "bright young guy—a keeper." I would cherish that epithet as one of the great understatements I have heard in my life. Even in that first week of getting to know him, I realized that he was just a bit beyond anyone else in his grasp of what went on in someone else's mind. That is why I was horrified when I had to present my first outpatient, Mr. D, to him. Paul savored the fine texture of emotions. My patient was catatonic. I had jabbered into Mr. D's icy, motionless stare for as long as I could stand it. Despite the assurance value of the patient's diagnosis, I was convinced that his unresponsiveness was a measure of my total lack of skill. To make matters worse, a sub rosa competition was going on in the intake group as to who could speak with insight and incisiveness worthy of Paul. More caught up in this declaiming contest than I realized, I transformed short happenings into long sentences. I cannot remember exactly now, but my text went something like, "Down the dimly lit corridor, dank with stale coffee odor, Mr. D and I lumbered toward our fateful encounter...." It was like that high-school report on the book one never quite read, an attempt to use see-through gloss to hide naked ignorance.

However, unlike any teacher I have ever had, Paul knew how to blot the overflow of shame with a powerful mixture of absorbents. He identified my dreaded state of mind, namely that I was really at a loss of words to match being at a loss of feelings. He credited me with nothing less than genius, because in not feeling anything I had clearly located the epicenter of Mr. D. He said nothing about what I should have done or could have said. Instead, he floated with the dilemma at hand: How was I to communicate to Paul, to the group, to Mr. D in the face of my identification with the breakdown of the most basic tie line of communication, the exchange of affect?

I, like so many others who knew Paul, was to have this unique experience of his containment again and again. In all the years of our friendship, the most blessed years of my life, I never caught on to the formula. Most other teachers I have loved and respected sooner or later betray the source of their magic. One can take in the Weltanschauung, the algorithm from which they work. With Paul, you almost could, but the "almost" is the critical word. Paul purposefully defied formula. As he states in the skiing analogy in these two papers, therapist and patient must locate together where prior injury, speed, the need to turn, the contour of the hill all coerce a missing competence. Paul defied formula because he was savvy enough to realize in the early 1970s that both patient and therapist could locate each other's prior injuries only to the extent that they together fell in and out of containment. The knowledge that mattered could be gained only after the fact (cf. Renik 1993). Paul defied formula because he demonstrated to all of us that to locate another required enormous struggle within oneself. Prior experience and mastery, as he says, allow us to fine tune the residual areas of affective incompetence.

With dedicated study we can "almost" take in Paul because he redefined the introject as an "almost." It is almost an algorithm, almost a representation of the way two people have been with each other, have corrected the past. However, it can never be complete. Each evocation of the Paul imago, of any imago, demands a reckoning with the uniqueness of who one is now and, in reflection, was then. To paraphrase Paul, the ultimate paradox is the sense of rediscovering what one has never before emotionally known.

PARADOX

Paul bore an intellectual kinship to Wittgenstein (1958), Rorty (1989), and certain postmodernists in the way that he helped us to see what is possible by defining the limits of seeing. However, in Paul's hands the very definition of constraint confers greater freedom. His own version of the intrinsic limits of emotional experience depends in particular on analogies based on his reading of Kuhn (1962), Quine (1976), and Gödel (1940). In many papers he turns to the barber paradox as a way of introducing a readership of mental-health professionals to the unexpected notion of a mathematics of competence. The barber paradox is both clear and "falsidical." There is no such person who can shave all and only those who cannot shave themselves, because he would then shave himself only if he didn't. The reason is simple: the premise is faulty. If our stickiest feeling dilemmas, like "is it me or is it you?", were like the barber paradox, we could resolve them by merely correcting mistaken logic (e.g., I falsely attribute my hatred to you).

However, Quine posits a thornier form of paradox, called an antinomy. For example, let us define the words that refer to themselves as autological and those that don't as heterological. In other words, "short" and "polynomial" are autological; "long" and "monosyllabic" are heterological. But what about "heterological?" If it refers to itself it is autological, and if it doesn't it is not "heterological." There is no clean way out, because the idea of words referring or not referring to themselves mostly escapes this dilemma. There is only one instance, the word "heterological," when things come to grief and not because of anything so simple as a false premise. As Paul pointed out, Betrand Russell's class of all classes that do not contain themselves as a member poses the same problem. Number theory would be consistent and complete if it did not have to deal with this one instance. This is the form of paradox that Quine called an antinomy.

PARADOX AND THE COGNITIVE FUNCTION OF AFFECT

Most students of the mind maintain a respectful wariness toward philosophers. After all, philosophers are the building inspectors of every other discipline's knowledge structures. They are employed to find the termites and faulty wiring. Paradox and antinomy are names applied to quaint vulnerabilities in certain thought structures that never really threatened their stability. Then came Kuhn (1962) and Gödel (1940). Each in his own way arrived at a disturbing truth: any attempt by the human mind to map a comprehensive theory will ultimately meet with grief. The very effort will sooner or later be confounded by paradox, the seeds of which were sown by the very attempt at consistency. Kuhn wrote about the crisis of confounding data that inevitably threatens a reigning scientific paradigm and occasions its overthrow by a better system of explanation. Gödel literally proved that any comprehensive theory of cardinal numbers would of necessity contain an inconsistency.

Paul brilliantly recognized that a person's emotional life is analogous to a paradigm or number theory. Because affect serves a cognitive function, the sum total of one's affective reactions maps an implicit view of the world of self and other. A person's very effort to frame this guiding view of why things feel as they do sows the seeds of inconsistency. The clearest example is that of the self-fulfilling prophecy. A patient insists that love leads to abandonment; there is no choice but to leave first. In the course of therapy, it becomes clear that leaving first leads to abandonment. Suddenly the patient is confronted with an agonizing uncertainty as to who actually leaves whom. Who is self and who is other? To Paul it was clear that the various meanings and action potentials of our feelings are ultimately caught in various antinomies of their own. He posited the existence of four essential types, illustrated in the form of rhetorical questions:

Is this me or is this you?
Did I do this or was it done to me?

Paradox and the Cognitive Function of Affect

Is this now or was it then?
Can I choose what I feel?

In one sense, all of Paul's writings are in content and style exercises in framing, savoring, and containing these several polarities that cannot be mutually reconciled. Repetition is the sameness in change. Perception is riddled with memory. Memory is riddled with perception (cf. Loewald 1980). The past is a construction of the present. However, in everyday life, we do not frame paradox in these abstract statements. Instead, we *sense* it in the greater or lesser moments of agony framed summarily by the rhetorical questions. I will offer a case example that in actuality is a composite of several treatment crises that I, Jane Grignetti, and Andrew Gill discussed with Paul at various points.

Mr. E, a patient for whom being understood is a prerequisite for existing, hears me recount how his doubts about a current woman in his life are linked to the bedrock of his suffering: growing up with a "dead mother" (cf. Green 1986). The specifics of what I said are lost to my memory. However, I do recall that I did not recognize anything in my words or myself at this time that countered the usual bounds of my empathy. What mattered was that the patient did. He said my grades had been pretty good up to that point, given his low expectations for any therapist. However, he now had deep suspicions that I was offering him some form of canned meat. He was panicked that I had lost him in revealing that I did not really know the nature of his hurt. Worst of all, he feared that I expected him to swallow my prepared meal, preservatives and all. I knew that his parents and others in his life had done just that to him. I also was momentarily sentient enough to embrace Paul's wise precept that this was no time for a speculation about the transference. Most of what went on between us in an escalating sequence of disjunctive moments could be readily captured by two of Paul's questions: "Is it you or is it me" and "Is it happening now or happening then?"

At the present time psychoanalysis has grown as a field, and we have a plethora of relevant theories that posit concepts more or less equivalent to Paul's ideas of repetition, relationship, affect, containment, and paradox. For instance, the vignette I described above was, depending on your theoretical outlook, an empathic failure, a "now moment," or an intersubjective disjunction. Take your pick. We can even say that many modernists (cf. Pizer 1996) have joined the ship that Paul launched so many years ago in believing that the crisis can be resolved only by genuine negotiation rather than authoritative interpretation. However, each of these seemingly equivalent ideas is usually defined by and allied with a body of technique. Once again, Paul sensed that the attempt to frame a comprehensive logic of therapeutic intervention would necessarily include its own fatal flaw, its region of incompetence. In other words, Paul extended Gödel's warning and suspected that a definitive set of techniques would bear a fate no different from that of a definitive theory of numbers.

Because he was resigned to the inevitability of paradox and paradigm shift, Paul could relish many aspects of just about every viewpoint within psychoanalysis. He enjoyed all theory, including his own, for what it could provide, namely the illusion that in the cool of the moment the treatment experience can be rendered into definitive description. But Paul was aware that once the heat is on, and the therapist is face to face with her patient, her theoretical introjects will expose their "almostness." At this point there is no choice except to leave them behind and enter the fray with that inchoate suit of armor known as *oneself*. The goal was a word he never wholly embraced: negotiation. He feared its being assimilated into his readers' images of business transactions. I think that he meant to imply the successful negotiation of a perilous turn in the slope of a relationship.

NEGOTIATION OF PARADOX

Was it me or was it him? I reiterate. That morning is hazy in recollection, and I do not know what I said to Mr. E. I retain the feel of my words and the afterglow of my intention. I felt I was myself. But who was I? I had and still have no idea; the patient had some. Of course, his wisdom was not certain either, but it was worth everything in its otherness. Paul parallels Lacan (1978) and Winnicott (1965) in his awareness that the inchoate edges of oneself exist only in the emotional reflections of another.

In addition, Paul cautions us again and again that the patient's inability to see anything as different from the way it was in the past is both a hard-won competence and a form of paranoia, that is, an area of affective incompetence. It is now a commonplace that the therapist is in a similar boat. Therapy, as it necessarily approaches its nadir, becomes the meeting of two areas of competence paradoxically contained in incompetence. "I *know* that I didn't say anything that bad!" I said something like that to myself as I tried to repair Mr. E's assault on the chainmail of my narcissism. And if I did, how bad was it? This thought was bathed in considerable shame and guilt. The rescue from this humiliation came from another turn in my mind: but, ah, the patient often feels that way, is defending against being wrong because of the fear he caused his mother's deadness! A moment of relief—all has been realigned—until I remember that I was feeling dead that morning. Dead tired (permissible, but barely so). Deadened by a somewhat annoying recognition that I am tired of having to reassure this patient of my presence (less permissible). Do I expiate my guilt with some kind of revelation to him of my generous *mea culpa*, or would my confession provide a rationale for punching Mr. E back with an overdose of awareness of his effect on me? Or do I sit still and contain this internal "gamoosh" (a Paul Russell term for chaos) and risk losing him some more as he becomes increasingly convinced that I cannot respond to him?

Paul, in my evocation of him, based on many actual moments now blended together in memory, modeled how one negotiates the profound, mutually fragmenting moments he called in his first paper "the crunch." Paradox courts urgency. Patient and therapist can hardly bear the legacy of the repetition compulsion, namely the sense that this sudden painful turn in the relationship has betrayed its potential lack of viability. Patient and therapist are threatened with various admixtures of failure and devastating aloneness. Paul once again absorbed the therapist's distress. He simply smiled and uttered in his most clipped "downeast" dialect some variant of his two pillars of clinical wisdom: "Damned if I know!" and "Just keep doing exactly what you are doing!" These two basic communiqués could be uttered in a variety of equivalences, like "How did you manage to come up with that! Brilliant!" or "Don't change a thing." I argued with him strenuously, and I know that others did as well. On occasion, I accused him of being incapable of criticism or confrontation. I told him that I needed it and, furthermore, could take it.

I missed the point. There was a complex method in his at times maddening kindness, which I eventually unpacked as follows. Paul, like Kohut, was steadfast in his belief that failure of recognition and the shame consequent to that failure were two of the most toxic pollutants in early development. At all costs, they were therefore to be contained in the treatment. He, like anyone in the role of supervisor, had a critical role in this containment. As a vehicle for containment, Paul would state again and again that the superego stood in lieu of competence. Always quick to think the best, he treated me as though I thoroughly understood him. Initially, I did not. Eventually, after a number of years of field experience in the ravages of my own compulsive repetitions, the meaning of this epigram began to dawn on me. Paul was onto how readily any of us in the field resort to an "I should" when we come face to face with certain critical ambiguities of relatedness. "I should be criticized" or "What should I do or say?" are both species of urgency that signal "I don't like what I feel right now." And not liking what one is feeling right now is, in turn, the necessary sign that genuine negotiation is in process. Paul's seemingly blanket encouragement was really a way of signaling me that a noisy conscience was a distraction from the necessity of savoring as much of one's bad feeling as one could. In a word, it was his hands-on method of coaching me in the vital skill of skiing to the edge of one's affective competence. The fall was never welcomed or graceful, but it was reliably instructive. As he states repeatedly in these two papers, each successive fall further defines the area of injury.

Mr. E's belief that I was handing him canned meat and my countering conviction that he had reasons for taking the freshness out of what I offered him were, for Paul, simultaneous translations of our respective reenacted traumas. Each of us in his own way took note, within the limits of our respective competence, of what had taken place. And each of us was necessarily constrained by what he could not yet feel. In other words, the degrees of freedom of what could be felt by either of us with regard to the other were determined by the dynamics of injury. Pain and initial inflammation are exaggerated, helpful, and delimiting responses. Healing, however, requires the recruitment of unknown intention inherent in what we are on the verge of feeling. The degrees of freedom of what could be felt, might have been felt, were slowly increased. Mr. E could and did realize in his recoil from my non-recognition an active intention to murder what recognition there was, to throw the food offered overboard as an angry statement that it was too little, too late. Or, he might and did relish tormenting me with his own form of non-recognition. I also began to have the disturbing realization that somewhere within me I felt the same way toward him.

AFFECT, EMERGENCE, AND DYNAMIC SYSTEMS

My description of how Mr. E and I negotiated and ultimately traversed a dangerous impasse could be viewed as an illustration of the role of projective identification as a defense against aggression. To whom did the angry self belong? The concept in its familiar connotation disposes us toward action, namely defense analysis: the patient *should* ultimately "fess up" that he left an unacceptable piece of himself in the therapist's storage locker. I note that the emphasis is on "should" and "fessing up," that is, on the responsibility of the patient to assume ownership. The injunction to analyse a defense often erodes into the temptation to prod or goad. In the example of the child who says the breast bit her, Paul makes a subtle yet crucial shift in the definition and implication of projective identification:

Paradox and the Cognitive Function of Affect

> We could, if we want, call her paranoid. But what is important here is something else. And that is that the little girl obviously needs her mother's breast right now in a specific and crucial way. The breast now serves as the receptacle, the container, for something belonging to the little girl that she cannot herself, right now, contain: that is, the wish to injure. [this volume, pp. 38–39]

Paul reminds us that the therapist's storage locker is really a safe-deposit box. The accent is shifted from pressing the patient to take ownership to understanding the patient's need to seek safekeeping. Unacceptable affects are to be placed in trust until therapist and patient achieve an integration in their relationship that restores the patient's capacity to feel. The patient will at that point be ready to take ownership.

Via the breast that bites, via all of his other declared myths and metaphors, Paul repeatedly and consistently shifts the emphasis of our most familiar modes of dynamic understanding. He turns our attention from instinct to affect, from defense to the capacity to feel, from acting out to intentionality. Paul Russell was like Hans Loewald in his brilliant ability to revolutionize psychoanalysis without the usual bloodshed. The landmarks of our past are preserved and cherished by at times radical restoration. As a result, if we manage to internalize Paul's ideas, we find that our clinical perspective has undergone a profound change. Therapeutic action, in Paul Russell's terms, consists of the effort to restore missing affective colorings simultaneously to the palettes of both patient and therapist. The clinical eye is to be first riveted on what can be seen, namely feeling tones, and not on what must be fantasied or inferred, for example, hierarchies of instincts and their vicissitudes. These metaphors are to be held in reserve as assists for an aerobics of the imagination, as he demonstrates for us in his workout with the death instinct. However, to return to "it bit me," the twists and turns of theory are most helpful when they point to ways in which we can expand the patient's capacity to feel—when they enhance the mathematics of competence.

It can be fairly said that Paul's thinking is itself no less than a theory. He indeed provided us with an outline for a calculus of affective interaction. However, as I stressed in the beginning, Paul differed from others by his acknowledgment that his understanding was "almost." He prepared us at every juncture for what is almost but never really known ahead of time. Paul was prescient in his awareness that the critical happenings of the treatment, be they defined as intrapsychic, intersubjective, or interactive, are not dictated by codes and patterns stored in an archival unconscious. Feeling and event *emerge* in the moment.

Paul's appreciation that key knowledge is emergent, contingent, and extrinsic was arrived at in stages. In the early '70s, he would often allude to Kant (1965) and the idea of the transcendental analytic. He was intrigued that foundational categories of knowledge might be intrinsic to the mind. However, as his focus turned specifically to the centrality of affect, he began to consolidate his idea that feelings mark the perimeter of what one is trying to know. Emotional understanding is extrinsic. Affects provide an essential orientation (cf. Lear 1990) toward the world by dint of their disposition and "aboutness" (cf. Dennett 1993). For example, the child *feels as though* the breast will bite her when she is angry *about* the birth of a sibling. Lastly, Paul challenged the tendency of all theorists since Freud to privilege one wish or motivation as primary. Paul accorded to each affect its own agenda and dominion within the mind.

The combination of all of these shifts in emphasis reconfigured our understanding of the bedrock of psychodynamic theory. I believe that, without using the term, Paul implicitly recast psychoanalysis as a dynamic systems theory. Thelen and Smith (1995) have accomplished the same goal with respect to various aspects of action and cognition. The case illustration they rely on is the development of walking in the infant. By carefully reviewing various strands of research, they make the radical statement that there is no central pattern generator or any other intrinsic program in the nervous system that guides and dictates motor development. As a matter of fact, all of human development is "soft assembled" rather than hard wired. In support of this thesis, Thelen and Smith convincingly demonstrate that the development of walking is based on the happenstance linkage of events similarly envisioned in chaos theory and the concept of parallel processing. From the mutual influence of environment, task, and various organismic subsystems (neurons and muscles in various states of excitement and position) there *emerge* complex patterns of limb motion. To say it simply, walking is determined not by a central committee of planning neurons but rather by the way the rubber meets the road. For environment, task, and organism, simply read hill, speed, and prior injury and it becomes evident why I believe Paul has given us a dynamical systems theory.

CONCLUSION

Paul Russell, Stern (1995), Thelen and Smith (1995), and other contemporary behavioral scientists share the common premise that we must let go of our belief that hypothetical ghosts in the machine account for what a person feels, thinks, and does.

According to contemporary developmental research, it is unlikely that preordained determinants within the person, for example, unconscious instinctual scripts, lead in predictable, linear fashion to the repetition compulsion. Instead, it is more likely that various tendencies and constraints operating in parallel from within the person and without, from within the relationship and without, combine in unpredictable fashion to repeat paradoxically what has never exactly happened before. In this version of how things work, there are many more degrees of freedom in the emotional life than have been postulated by any prior theory. In a word, neither the unconscious, character, nor drive is truly destiny. Instead, as Paul states, "the treatment process discovers the feelings and the injury to them. . . . The affect sculpts out exactly the problem of relatedness that has not yet been solved" (pp. 45–46). I would add that affect also sculpts out the definition of the problem which does not exist until then. Paul's honesty about what therapy was not enhanced its potential to be more than we ever thought it could be. His most beguiling metaphor invokes the healing process. It is not something that can be either micromanaged or second guessed. But if we safeguard the conditions that allow it to happen, it will work of its own inchoate and often miraculous accord.

REFERENCES

Dennett, D. (1993). *The Intentional Stance.* Cambridge, MA: MIT Press.

Gödel, K. (1940). *The Consistency of the Continuum Hypothesis.* Princeton: Princeton University Press.

Green, A. (1986). *On Private Madness.* Madison, CT: International Universities Press.

Kant, I. (1965). *Critique of Pure Reason.* Trans. N. K. Smith. New York: St. Martin's.

Kuhn, T. S. (1962). *The Structure of Scientific Revolutions.* Chicago: University of Chicago Press.

Lacan, J. (1978). *The Four Fundamental Concepts of Psycho-Analysis.* New York: Norton.

Lear, J. (1990). *Love and Its Place in Nature.* New York: Farrar, Straus, and Giroux.

Loewald, H. (1980). Perspectives on memory. In *Papers on Psychoanalysis*, pp. 96–114. New Haven, CT: Yale University Press.

Pizer, S. (1996). Negotiating potential space: illusion, play, metaphor, and the subjunctive. *Psychoanalytic Dialogues* 6:689–712.

Quine, W. V. (1976). *The Ways of Paradox and Other Essays.* Cambridge, MA: Harvard University Press.

Renik, O. (1993). Analytic interaction: conceptualizing technique in the light of the analyst's irreducible subjectivity. *Psychoanalytic Quarterly* 62:553–571.

Rorty, R. (1989). *Contingency, Irony, and Solidarity.* New York: Cambridge University Press.

Stern, D. N. (1995). *The Motherhood Constellation.* New York: Basic Books.

Thelen, E., and Smith, L. B. (1995). *A Dynamic Systems Approach to the Development of Cognition and Action.* Cambridge, MA: MIT Press/Bradford Books.

Tomkins, S. (1962). *Affect, Imagery, Consciousness*, vol. 1. New York: Springer.

Winnicott, D. W. (1965). *The Maturational Processes and the Facilitating Environment.* New York: International Universities Press.

Wittgenstein, L. (1958). *Philosophical Investigations.* New York: Macmillan.

SEVEN

UNDERSTANDING REPETITION AND THE TREATMENT CRISIS: A VIEW OF PAUL RUSSELL'S THEORETICAL ORIENTATION

Jane H. Leavy, LICSW

Let me recapitulate one final time. Our patients come to us in a crisis. They may not define it, or even feel it as such. But the very fact that they have sought us out says that there is something that they feel unable to do on their own. We have to assume that had they been able to do it on their own, they would have long since done it. They bring to us an organization of all that they have been able to do so far; and they bring to us as well, equally well organized, that which they have been *unable* to do on their own. The repetition compulsion is an organized system of affective incompetence. It is a confusion of memory and desire, memory representing itself as desire. The organization, the intelligence, of the repetition compulsion consists of the invitation, however muted, to attachment. It may take a little time for us to get a feel for what exactly that is. And we might not get it quite right the first time. Or the second. Or the third. We may never know precisely what happened. What we can know, however, is that patients may find us safe enough to deliver the most dangerous parts of their lives.

We begin to *feel* what it is that is dangerous. This turns out to be much better, much more useful information than the most precise historical knowledge. Our patients' repetitions with us are highly organized, refined distillations of what, emotionally, they are unable to do on their own. Repetitions are functional, not necessarily historical, although the actual history is relevant. Repetition is delivered as a crisis, a crisis of attachment, where we are invited to *detach* [emphasis added], perhaps because we might need to, at precisely the point where, had someone been there, the repetition would not be necessary for either party.

If the therapist can feel the need to detach as information as opposed to urgency, it is possible to understand something emotionally that would not have happened otherwise. The restitution, the compensation, cannot ever happen, cannot ever take place, by anyone, for anyone. Both therapist and patient have spent time together trying to not know this. The only real restitution is grief. But it is a grief that makes the past real, and the present realizable. Grief makes possible a boundary, a new boundary between the past and the present, the capacity to remember then and desire now. [Russell 1994]

Paul Russell was a teacher and a practitioner of psychoanalysis who belonged to no one school of analytic theory. His way of thinking and his way of being were joined in his particular, personal stance and view of the analytic situation. Certain ideas, like that of the repetition compulsion, illuminated what he saw that patients presented, but his response to what he saw, what he thought analysis *was*, was very much his own creation. While always cautioning against a defensive over-attachment to theory, he also depended on theory to help him understand the clinical encounter.

Russell once wrote that he spoke about the repetition compulsion "repetitively [and] compulsively" (1988, p. 119). It was an idea to which he referred, over and over again, to understand why people, over and over again, repeat experiences that are painful and presumably ones they would rather not have repeated. "Affective incompetence," the necessity to repeat arising in the wake of a failure to feel, is the problem, he argued. And in his logical, mathematical way, he stated his theorem that "the capacity to feel has its origin, always, in a relationship. The corollary to this would be that interruptions in the development of the capacity to feel represent interruptions in relationships. . . . [T]he repetition compulsion represents the interruption of some important early relationship. [It is] the scar tissue of the injury to the capacity to feel" (p. 129).

In the passage cited at the beginning of this paper, Russell summarizes his working theory of the repetition compulsion in the context of the clinical encounter. He points to a particular phenomenon that occurs during a crisis or impasse in a therapy, namely the delivery of grief, grief that belongs historically to early ruptures in attachment and contains the core affects of sadness, rage, hopelessness, and shame that repeatedly emerge in moments of disrupted relatedness at critical times in life. It is grief, however, that cannot be borne in the present and cannot be understood to belong to the past. Grief is transformed into urgency, the urgent necessity to act, or to make the therapist act, to stop the feeling. The crisis in therapy is felt by both patient and therapist as occurring in the present, but it bears uncanny similarities to crises in the patient's life in the past. These eruptions of grief, and the unendurable affects that the grief contains, sometimes leave the patient and the therapist close to the brink of a rupture not unlike what may have occurred in the original traumatic breakdown of an attachment. So the experience repeats, and the treatment relationship is threatened. And, of course, grief is not the sole property of the patient. Contained in treatment crises are repetitions by the therapist of interruptions of relatedness in her life as well. It is, however, the job of the therapist to contain her urgent impulse to act, to try to avoid rupturing the safety of the containing treatment. The patient may need to do; the therapist needs to feel and to understand.

For Russell, the theory of the repetition compulsion functioned as a compass. While operating paradoxically, leading both patient and therapist to believe they must act, not feel, it nevertheless functioned to orient him during a crisis when the treatment felt as though it had lost its direction, and it instructed him in the meanings of the intense affect aroused in both people. The *fact* of the repetition compulsion, in all of its terrifying inevitability, is both what makes therapy curative and what makes it dangerous. The *theory* of the repetition compulsion provides a containing and orienting guide for the therapist, and, by implication, for the process.

What follows is an attempt, albeit sketchy and one that could never do justice to the originality and creativity of Russell's mind, to suggest what I think is Russell's particular contribution to psychoanalytic thinking, to place it on the historical continuum in which he thought and wrote and supervised, in a sense to place his work on the map of psychoanalytic writing. This particular selection of psychoanalytic neighbors among which to place Paul is entirely my own.

As I see it, the psychoanalytic traditions among which Russell's writing belongs range between classical, Freudian theory and modern theories of trauma and affect. He was loyal to the timeless wisdom and compelled by the rich metaphors of Freud's writing, but he also saw it as a product of its own culture and Freud's own positivistic scientific philosophy. The fundamental importance of attachment, which John Bowlby argued was the central ethological force that preceded drive, appears to be something Russell simply assumed was true.

Russell's ideas are compatible with those of Hans Loewald and Arnold Modell, two important writers who link the generations of psychoanalysts. His elliptical, sometimes epigrammatic style and his love of paradox are reminiscent of Donald Winnicott. His approach to understanding the patient is close to that of one of his own teachers, Elvin Semrad. His thinking is very close to new theories of development, particularly those growing out of infant research and emphasizing the centrality of affect and affective communication. New research that demonstrates the centrality of early attachment experience in the laying down of lifelong affective and relational patterning seems to confirm Russell's view of repetition. However, he took exception to what he felt were the excesses of the intersubjectivists, in that he disagreed with the notion that we really can know or join with the other's subjectivity, while granting always the influence of the other's affect on our own subjective reality. And lastly, Russell's view of the determining and controlling influence of trauma and unendurable grief is very similar to the thinking of contemporary trauma theorists such as Judith Herman and Bessel van der Kolk, and of writers who have studied holocaust survivors and their families, in that Russell pointed to the crippling impact of trauma that moves silently through lifetimes, through relationships, and through succeeding generations.

FREUD, BOWLBY, AND LOEWALD

Russell's use of the concept of the repetition compulsion links his thought to Freud's in "Remembering, repeating, and working-through" (1914) and *Beyond the Pleasure Principle* (1920) and at the same time places him in the category of psychoanalytic revisionist. Freud (1920) argued that the existence of the repetition compulsion was proof of the existence of the death instinct. He used the repetitive phenomena he observed in traumatic war neuroses and in children's play to further his metapsychology and psychology of instinct. The death instinct, he argued, is a force that grows out of "the conservative nature of living substance," and he pointed to the tendency in organic life "toward the restoration of an earlier state of things" (pp. 36–37). Freud's view was that biologically and psychologically there is instinctual movement toward death throughout life, as part of our heredity.

It is possible, however, to separate the ideas of repetition and instinct, to see the repetition compulsion as a clinically observable phenomenon, while understanding the notion of the death instinct metaphorically. This seems to have been Russell's compromise. The metaphor of the death instinct, not understood literally, directs our attention to what Freud calls the "daemonic" (1933, p. 107) nature of repetitions, their "malignancy" in Russell's words, and their origins, which Russell traced directly to trauma.

In a paper he gave at Swarthmore College in 1990, Russell grappled with the question of trauma, what he referred to as the psychology of event relating to the fact of real-life trauma, and the psychology of intention relating to the psychoanalytic theory of intrapsychic conflict and wish. He decided on the paradoxical probability of both being true, but in a particular way: "the mark of trauma is the retroactive sense of having intended it. Patients have a glimpse that this is not true—they did not intend that which injured them, at least not in the first instance—but to face that down confronts them with a loss, a loss that carries with it an unendurable white-hot pain. It amounts to a loss of their past" (1990 , p. 137). And so people repeat, and do not know which came first, what was done to them or what they appear to be doing to themselves.

Russell's revision of Freud takes us to the idea of trauma instead of to the death instinct, pointing us to event instead of intention, and back to intention again. The repetition compulsion is the proof of trauma, of early injury to the capacity to feel, and it is therefore as dangerous to life as a death instinct would be. We could argue that the residue of trauma amounts to a death-instinct equivalent: "insofar as one is traumatized, insofar as one repeats the past, insofar as one hates, to that extent one murders time, one does not choose, does not act, does not live. In other words, trauma, the repetition compulsion, the wish to kill, illness, and the sapping of energies of life, are intimately bound together" (this volume, p. 43).

Russell's agreement with Freud is in some sense more important than his disagreement. In his own time, and within the limits of his own biological theory, Freud's discovery was remarkable. He noticed that patients repeated "experiences which include no possibility of pleasure," and in studying patients with war neuroses and recurring traumatic dreams, he hypothesized "a time before the purpose of dreams was the fulfillment of wishes" (1920, pp. 36–37). This "time before" represents a state in which experience is not laid down in memory but belongs to the not-remembered, affectively organized layer of experience that is left imprinted by traumatic events. Some part of traumatic experience is encoded in the brain, giving rise to a compulsion to repeat, recreate, and reenact that which can "include no possibility of pleasure," or, as Russell would say, "something one would far rather not repeat" (undated, p. 3).

By dating the origins of the repetition compulsion back to the earliest relationships and to disturbances of attachment, Russell is implicitly referring to the work of John Bowlby (1960). Bowlby took the position that interruptions of attachment by separation in the first two years of life lead to grief and mourning in children, and potentially to impairment in later object relations. In papers and films, Bowlby demonstrated the deep and lasting injurious effects on children of traumatic separations or ruptures of the attachment process. And, over the course of his life, Bowlby developed an instinct theory of his own, one that placed attachment at the biologically determined center of development, positing that it is in the attachment process that the child develops the capacity to regulate affect, and that interruptions in attachment lead to grief even in a very young child. This perhaps is the "time before," when the original impressions of love and attachment, hate and loss occur and leave their mark on the developing personality for the rest of life. By referring to disruptions of attachment, Russell implicitly placed the greatest vulnerability to trauma, and therefore to injuries that lead to unconscious repetition, in the earliest years of life. My sense, however, is that he used the term *attachment* loosely as well, referring not just to trauma in the first two years but also to ruptures in connection and trust or dependency at many points in the life cycle, ruptures that later lead to unbidden repetition.

Hans Loewald's seminal paper "On the therapeutic action of psychoanalysis" was published in 1960, in the same year that Bowlby's paper on grief and mourning was published. Freud's language of death and death instinct is echoed in Loewald's writing about the nature of transference repetition. But Loewald's paper represents a complicated juncture of a number of psychoanalytic ideas of that time, in that he writes in the idiom of classical instinct theory and ego psychology but recasts psychoanalytic ideas into a relational framework by way of his concept of internalization. Citing Freud's reference to the *Odyssey* in *The Interpretation of Dreams*, he speaks of "ghosts which awoke to new life as soon as they tasted blood," referring to the revival of deep unconscious memory of early relationships at the moment of opportunity in the transference. He writes, wryly but evocatively, that "those who know ghosts tell us that they long to be released from their ghost life and led to rest as ancestors. As ancestors they live forth in the present generation with their shadow life" (p. 249). Therapy, and in particular the transference, is the medium of this change, the ghosts of the past no longer haunting the patient but enriching the patient's life as ancestors. Loewald points to the creative possibility of transference, where a new relationship is forged out of old internalizations awakened and transformed. Without recreations of this kind, he writes, "human life becomes sterile and an empty shell" (p. 250).

I would argue that Loewald and Russell shared a view of the nature of repetition and the nature of treatment. Loewald, who writes of the analyst's "love and respect for the individual and for individual development" (p. 229), worried that he would be misunderstood by his generation of analysts who adhered strictly to principles of objective, scientific neutrality in the analyst (E. Loewald 1994). So we see in Loewald a certain compromise, a stance in which an abstaining analyst communicates love implicitly by refraining from repeating early object ties.

But it is in the relationship with the analyst, and the affect roused in that relationship, that change occurs: "When it comes to the transference repetitions, it is as though the differentiation of past and present—one of the crucial advances in early psychic development—has to be undertaken all over again. We know that this differentiation tends to recede in proportion to the increasing intensity of affect even in recollective remembering" (H. Loewald, 1975, p. 359). While it was ideologically radical to propose this at the time, Loewald was clearly pointing to the extent to which analysis, at its deepest, is the crucible in which old experiences, by way of repetition, are transformed, and stating that the possibility for this transformation originates in the affective exchange between patient and analyst, not in the solitary inner psyche of the patient, aided only by the analyst's interpretations.

Loewald writes of the close link between memory and mourning, and in his paper "Perspectives on memory" (1976) points to the restitutive possibilities of memory, and, by implication, of repetition: "The past would be irretrievably lost without memory; in fact there would not be any past, just as there would not be any present that has meaning or any future to envisage. The fact that memory lets us have a past means that we experience loss and the irretrievability of the past and yet can recover the past in another form" (p. 148). Later in the same paper he speaks of "enactive and representational remembering." In the former the past and present are indistinguishable, and in the latter "the mind presents something to itself as its own past experience." He goes on to note that "any significant degree of affect present in representational remembering brings it closer to reenactment" (pp. 164–165). So memory and affect are joined, repetition and reenactment are the implied risk, mourning occurs, and restitution, possibly, is gained. This is very close to Paul Russell's thinking about grief, in that Loewald links the inevitability of repetition and enactment to the problem of loss and mourning and to the possibility of hope for the future. Loewald and Russell both saw that hope as residing in the treatment relationship.

WINNICOTT AND MODELL

D. W. Winnicott writes about these matters in his own particular style, approaching the problem of trauma, repetition, and affective exchange between patient and analyst with questions that I think are similar to those Loewald was trying to answer, and that Russell grappled with. Winnicott, however, unlike Loewald, does not try to resolve the paradoxes inherent in these areas by turning to a structural model. Instead he illuminates paradoxes and gives them a home in the form of the transitional space, the area between illusion and reality, in which psychoanalytic transactions are conducted. In this space it is possible for patient and analyst to live in the past and the present simultaneously, and for affective exchange to occur in all its deep and risky complexity and yet be contained. The transitional space is the heir to the original mother–baby relationship and as such must be creative and elastic enough to tolerate intense exchanges of love and hate.

Winnicott argues strenuously in "Hate in the countertransference" (1947) for the admissability of hate in the analyst, particularly in the treatment of psychotic patients. He speaks of "objective hate," hate the patient seems to provoke, as hate that is, paradoxically, the sign of the possibility of love. And so it is essential, if the patient is ever to experience the analyst's love, that the analyst know, and not retreat from, his own hate. Here

Winnicott is talking about negotiation of affect, an idea Russell elaborated. Russell saw this negotiation of intense feelings, including the exchange of love and hate, as central to the process of working through a treatment impasse.

In "Fear of breakdown" (1963) Winnicott postulates that the memory of "primitive agonies" constitutes a form of resistance in therapy, a form described as "fear of a breakdown that has already been experienced" (pp. 89–90). Again he holds us in this ambiguous space between then and now, illusion and reality, while he illuminates the terror that binds repetitions in their static, unyielding position. The certainty that the trauma is about to occur in the treatment is equivalent to a memory of a trauma that has already happened and that, in Russell's language, awaits rendering. There is the possibility, in the safety of the therapeutic relationship in which love and hate and terror and doubt can all be felt by both people, that a new kind of breaking down can occur, in a setting that does not belong to the past, and in preparation for new growth.

Arnold Modell expands on Winnicott's concept of the holding environment, both writers seeing this all-important maternal environment as represented in the day-to-day structure of the treatment relationship and arguing that this structure is an aspect, albeit a silent one in most circumstances, of the therapeutic action. Modell's view is that this idea is particularly relevant in understanding the treatment of narcissistic patients, whose capacity for relatedness to the analyst is impaired as a result of early failures of maternal holding. These failures of holding are the equivalent of the ruptures of attachment that Russell writes about. In a bold statement that separates him from his ego-psychological colleagues, Modell (1984) argues that treatment represents a possibility for return to that early experience of failure and for new development to occur in patients with significant character disturbances. He also takes the position that symbolic communication through language is not necessarily the primary vehicle of therapeutic interaction: *"we would say that the patient's affects are the transmitter of data, and the transmission only occurs when there is an affect bond between the patient and the observing analyst"* (p. 160, emphasis in original). Here, as for Russell, affect is the medium of analytic communication. Modell (1990) also elaborates on Winnicott's idea that treatment takes place in a transitional space somewhere between illusion and reality. He stresses the importance of understanding the multiple, paradoxical levels of reality in the treatment setting, which have no equivalent in ordinary life. It is this paradoxical quality that gives rise to a list of questions Russell posed in a number of his papers: "Is this me, or is this you? Is this now, or was it then? Did I do this, or was it done to me? Can I choose what I feel?" (this volume, p. 8). The question "is this now, or was it then?" can only be answered: it is both.

It is in this phenomenon, the dynamic relationship between past and present, linked by affect and experienced as memory in the present, that the repetition compulsion originates, as does the opportunity for transference to occur, for old and new to meet, and for therapeutic action to unfold. Modell and others see this way of understanding treatment as absolutely crucial in work with more acutely troubled patients. In *Other Times, Other Realities* Modell takes a position very close to Russell's view of repetition: "what is stored in memory is not a replica of the event, but rather the *potential* to generalize or refind the category or class of which the event is a member. . . . [T]o the extent that a given affect category represents unassimilated trauma, or a central pathogenic fantasy, there will be a pressure to evoke a corresponding countertransference affective response in the other person that will be self-confirming." These moments involve "a perceptual identity between past and present . . . [so that] repetition of affects is a self-fulfilling prophecy" (1990, pp. 64–65).

An important recent debate in psychoanalysis has been about whether the analyst is more or less an innocent bystander in the fulfilling of the patient's traumatic prophecy. To what degree does the analyst contribute to the rising affective tide, particularly during treatment crises? Infant research by Stern (1985), Beebe and Lachmann (1994), and others suggests that the very same mode of exchange that exists between infants and caregivers in the earliest weeks of life, the system whereby all of us learn to feel and to register the feelings of the other, is brought into the treatment relationship. The implication is that the affective overlay or underlay of each action of the therapist, including her interpretations, contributes significantly to the meaning made by the patient of that action. Likewise, the analyst takes in all of the affective charge of the patient's words and actions, and her actions are in some sense shaped by the meanings she makes of that charge.

In trying to understand the implications of these ideas for a theory of treatment, Modell, I think, would come down on the side of the more traditional view that the patient, by means of projective identification, draws the analyst into the repetition and creates the conditions for the analyst to fulfill the prophecy. The patient's past and the affect associated with it essentially drive the treatment. Modell sees it as the analyst's job to preserve the therapeutic frame by means of interpretation, to remain observing more than participating. Russell would place himself more on the side of a dynamic, interactive, or relational view, seeing himself as being available for participation in the patient's repetition via his own potential for repetition, or as being at least as susceptible as anyone else to the power of affect and its urgency. Interpretation may be what the analyst does while attempting to understand and while resisting the impulse to act rather than feel. Interpretation is important insofar as it helps the analyst understand, but Russell regarded interpretation as primarily the container of the analyst's affect, while both patient and analyst try to wait out the tide.

THEORIES OF AFFECT AND INTERSUBJECTIVITY

Russell's idea that treatment impasses recapitulate early ruptures of attachment, ruptures that produced a disorganizing and deregulating of affect, a loss of connection, and grief, is compatible with contemporary thinking about mutual influence in affective development in the parent–infant dyad. His views are similar to those of Daniel Stern (1985) and other developmentalists who have demonstrated the ways that interactions between babies and caregivers are encoded and generalized in the form of procedural memory and come to form a relational template in the developing child. Recent neurobiological findings by Allan Schore (1994) support these theories of the lasting and repetitive nature of early interactional and attachment experiences.

In contrast, however, Russell resisted the view of the intersubjectivists that *everything* in analysis is best understood as mutually regulated, and in doing so he allied himself with certain traditional constructs and metaphors belonging more to a one-person psychology, like the repetition compulsion and the death instinct, which he found illuminating if not necessarily fully explanatory. In an uncharacteristically aggressive way, Russell (1995) fiercely objected to positions taken by Robert Stolorow in his theory of intersubjectivity, a theory that has grown out of infant research and the self-psychology movement. Yet Stolorow's views on the centrality of affect and the relationship between trauma and psychopathology are very close to Russell's. Stolorow states that "the essence of trauma lies in the experience of unbearable affect" (Stolorow and Atwood 1992, p. 52) and goes on to argue that unbearable affect occurs in the context of a relationship. It usually originates in a relationship between a child and caregiver that has broken down, in which attunement has failed, the equivalent again of a rupture of attachment. The organization and disorganization of this early system of attachment and attunement are carried forward in life and reevoked and repeated in later relationships. Stolorow's theory of ruptured attachment and the inevitability of retraumatization, including in the treatment, is very similar to Russell's.

Russell's objection to Stolorow's theory centers more on the problem of its claim than on its content. To Russell, Stolorow's view that treatment involves an intersubjective, as opposed to an "interaffective," negotiation fails because it presumes a degree of empathy he did not think possible. He writes: "it is our feelings, not our subjectivities that connect us, both to other people and ourselves" (1995, p. 3). Subjectivity consists of affects and meanings arranged in utterly original ways; it is to be discovered but cannot ever be fully known by, or in any way cloned in, another person. He therefore regards the reifying of an "intersubjectivity" or space in which subjectivities meet as inherently contradictory, and therefore a theory of treatment that presupposes this space as suspect.

It seems that Russell was responding to a theory of affect and mutuality that he agreed with, joined to a theory of therapeutic action that he did not agree with. Taken together, Stolorow's position was so sweeping and so ponderous that Russell believed it would inevitably lead the struggling analyst away from the heart of the matter, namely the feelings in her or in the patient. Russell used this opportunity to state a central point about theory making: "the issue, here, is not where to locate, unremittingly, the ultimate constitutive matrix of psychological reality. The issue is the terror that can arise whenever one attempts to locate what is real" (1995, p. 4). Once again, Russell is noticing that the danger to the treatment can lie in the analyst's resistance to what either she or the patient feels. That resistance can be embedded in theory itself and in the analyst's attachment to her theory when she seeks protection from the patient's disturbing affect.

SEMRAD

Russell, in this discussion and elsewhere, echoes one of his own teachers, Elvin Semrad, whose theory of treatment lives on among his many students in a volume of quotations (Rako and Mazer 1983). Semrad had a unique working theory of therapeutic practice that was never codified and as a result seems almost livelier than some theories that were. It was Semrad's view that sadness and grief are at the heart of the matter in psychotherapy. It is in locating these deepest affects, and giving them opportunity for expression, that therapy does its work. Semrad is quoted as saying that "a man's either scared, mad, or sad. If he's talking about anything else, he's being superficial" (p. 115). And, referring to the therapist whose theory might eclipse the patient, he warned that "the only truth you have is your patient. And the only thing that interferes with that truth is your own perception. You may not be free to observe what is there to be observed, chiefly because it evokes feelings in you that are so troublesome that you quit looking" (p. 112). Semrad saw psychosis as a retreat from unbearable affect, a refusal to feel what is really happening, a retreat that is necessitated by infantile experiences of unbearable rupture or loss (Harvey Mazer, personal communication). In this sense, psychosis is only an extreme position taken in response to a universal, profoundly hazardous, aspect of life. Semrad and Russell saw psychosis as both containing the material, the grief, derived from the early rupture of attachment and also operating as a defense against knowledge of that rupture or that grief.

TRAUMA THEORY AND THE HOLOCAUST

Throughout Paul Russell's writing there are implicit underlying references to contemporary theories of trauma (see also Herman 1992, van der Kolk 1987). Russell regarded both early trauma and trauma in adult life as having the power to overwhelm affect and perception and to freeze the past enduringly and repetitively on the present. He agreed with trauma theorists that so-called "borderline" phenomena are derivative of trauma and argued that the core of the treatment is the effort to preserve the relationship against the inevitable repetitions (1989). So he takes trauma theory one large step further, in stressing the patient's need for a new relationship, one in which the therapist can *feel* the trauma and live through new iterations of the traumatic experience with the patient, including ones delivered directly into the treatment in the form of an impasse, a psychosis or psychotic transference, or any crisis that threatens to overwhelm the relationship. Facing down a history of trauma, in Russell's view, brings us inevitably into traumatic experiences with our patients and into periods when we can feel the dread, the rage, the insult, the horror, and the grief. Trauma theorists point to the countertransference resistance in the therapist to hearing the sometimes gruesome, terrifying stories of their patients' experiences. Russell argues that it may not be as important to know all the details as it is to know the feelings, and that patients recognize when their therapist can or cannot bear to do that. In very moving accounts of treatments with holocaust survivors and their children (Bergmann 1982, Herzog 1982) we hear of the silent transmission of unmetabolized trauma over the course of generations and of the power of psychotherapy to break that chain. To Russell, the actual events, which in the case of the children of survivors occurred to other people and before the patients were born, represent only the tip of the trauma. Silently, wordlessly, the trauma repeats by feel, encroaching always on new experiences, on new lives, always defining the present by the fear of, in Winnicott's (1963) language, the breakdown that has already happened. It is the work of treatment to alter this malignant course, and that occurs by making available the possibility of an attachment.

CONCLUSION

Psychoanalytic theories that place trauma, affect, attachment, and reenactment at the heart of the treatment process place the older principles of analytic assymetry and neutrality at risk (Fishman 1996, Renik 1993). Paul Russell thought and wrote on this theoretical edge. There are dangers involved for both patient and therapist in the discovery of deep unconscious wells of affect linked to early ruptures in attachment and to trauma, dangers that are inevitably encountered in the intimacy of the psychotherapeutic relationship, and in particular in the so-called "difficult treatment." These dangers are equaled only by the essential value and life-giving possibilities that such discovery may permit. Structural models developed by earlier generations of psychoanalysts are very useful in enabling an analyst to think, but they may not help her feel what is emerging from the patient. Russell, along with many contemporary writers, argues that it is in the emergence of feeling in both the patient and the analyst, and the affective exchange between them, that the healing properties of psychoanalysis reside. Russell's unique contribution, however, lies in the way he moved among these theoretical traditions, orienting himself in a classical Freudian construct, the repetition compulsion, while reinventing it in modern relational terms. Russell wove together aspects of several generations of psychoanalytic thinking that he found illuminating and enduring, and that he believed made it possible to grasp some of the most troubling events encountered in a psychotherapy.

Paul Russell (1995) observed that "our theories are our love objects. There is almost nothing an analyst is more passionate about than his theory. The reason is, I think, that we need our theories to bind our terror." Russell was widely respected as a teacher as well as a supervisor and consultant, particularly in the situation of the difficult treatment, yet consultations with him rarely involved discussion of psychoanalytic theory. He was known and trusted in the community as someone to turn to in the midst of a treatment crisis, or the "crunch," as he called it. He was someone who could grasp the "feel" of a terrible moment in a patient's life or in the life of a treatment, and someone who could steady a shaken therapist enough to enable him or her to resume helping the patient. In hindsight it is clear that he relied deeply on his understanding of the nature of repetition: its universality, its inevitability, its dangers to the patient, the therapist, and the treatment, and its potential for healing, to guide him and sustain his compassionate receptivity to the painful and difficult matters that emerge in a treatment crisis. He was unfailingly steady, kind, and thoughtful, respectful of both therapist and patient, and profoundly committed to the work of therapy even at its most difficult and risky. Theory was perhaps present in discussions, but operating in the background, never used to justify a position taken, never eclipsing the intensity of the feelings in the treatment. His writing, highly theoretical in its own way, reflects this balance, in that we can always hear his voice and sense his presence, arguing for the personal before the theoretical, understanding the necessity to turn to theory to orient ourselves, and warning against our tendency to love our theories too much. His writing, which belongs among the writing of other important teachers in psychoanalysis, is his lasting contribution to those who did not know him, and of some comfort and an abiding inspiration to those who did.

REFERENCES

Beebe, B., and Lachmann, F. (1994). Representation and internalization in infancy: three principles of salience. *Psychoanalytic Psychology* 2:127–165.

Bergmann, M. (1982). Recurrent problems in the treatment of survivors and their children. In *Generations of the Holocaust*, ed. M. Bergmann and M. Jucovy, pp. 247–266. New York: Basic Books.

Bowlby, J. (1960). Grief and mourning in infancy. *Psychoanalytic Study of the Child* 15:9–52. New York: International Universities Press.

Fishman, G. (1996). Listening to affect: interpersonal aspects of affective resonance in psychoanalytic treatment. In *Understanding*

Therapeutic Action: Psychodynamic Concepts of Cure, ed. L. Lifson, pp. 217–235. Hillsdale, NJ: Analytic Press.

Freud, S. (1914). Remembering, repeating, and working-through. *Standard Edition* 12:145–156.

——— (1920). Beyond the pleasure principle. *Standard Edition* 18:3–64.

——— (1926). Inhibitions, symptoms and anxiety. *Standard Edition* 20:77–175.

——— (1933). New introductory lectures. *Standard Edition* 22:3–182.

Herman, J. (1992). *Trauma and Recovery.* New York: Basic Books.

Herzog, J. (1982). World beyond metaphor. In *Generations of the Holocaust,* ed. M. Bergmann and M. Jucovy, pp. 103–119. New York: Basic Books.

Loewald, E. (1994). *Introductory Remarks.* Paper presented at the Massachusetts Institute for Psychoanalysis Symposium on Therapeutic Action, Cambridge, MA, October.

Loewald, H. (1960). On the therapeutic action of psychoanalysis. In *Papers on Psychoanalysis,* pp. 221–256. New Haven, CT: Yale University Press, 1980.

——— (1975). Psychoanalysis as an art, and the fantasy character of the psychoanalytic situation. In *Papers,* pp. 352–371.

——— (1976). Perspectives on memory. In *Papers,* pp. 148–173.

Modell, A. (1984). *Psychoanalysis in a New Context.* Madison, CT: International Universities Press.

——— (1990). *Other Times, Other Realities.* Cambridge, MA: Harvard University Press.

Rako, S. and Mazer, H. (1983). *Semrad, the Heart of a Therapist.* New York: Jason Aronson.

Renik, O. (1993). Analytic interaction: conceptualizing technique in light of the analyst's irreducible subjectivity. *Psychoanalytic Quarterly* 62:553–571.

Russell, P. (1988). The search for safety. Unpublished paper.

——— (1989). On the diagnosis and treatment of the borderline. Paper presented at Boston Psychoanalytic Society and Institute, Boston, MA, April.

——— (1990). Trauma, repetition, affect. Unpublished paper.

——— (1994). The risk of psychotherapy. Paper presented at Cambridge Hospital, Cambridge, MA, April.

——— (1995). Discussion of the intersubjective perspective. Paper presented at Symposium on the Therapeutic Action of Psychodynamic Psychotherapy, Boston, MA.

——— (undated). The compulsion to repeat. Unpublished paper.

Schore, A. (1994). *Affect Regulation and the Origin of the Self: The Neurobiology of Emotional Development*. Hillsdale, NJ: Lawrence Erlbaum.

Stern, D. (1985). *The Interpersonal World of the Infant*. New York: Basic Books.

Stolorow, R., and Atwood, G. (1992). *Contexts of Being: The Intersubjective Foundations of Psychological Life*. Hillsdale, NJ: Analytic Press.

van der Kolk, B. (1987). *Psychological Trauma*. Washington, DC: American Psychiatric Press.

Winnicott, D. W. (1947). Hate in the countertransference. In *Through Paediatrics to Psycho-analysis*, pp. 194–203. New York: Basic Books, 1975.

——— (1963). Fear of breakdown. In *Psychoanalytic Explorations*, ed. C. Winnicott, R. Shepard, and M. Davis, pp. 87-95. Cambridge, MA: Harvard University Press.

INDEX

Action
  cognition and affect and, 34–36
  and memory, 61–62
  motivation for, 80–82
  patient's need for, 125–126
Affect, 11, 38–39. *See also* Affective competence; Affective incompetence
  capacity for, 7, 19–21, 32, 45–46, 74
  and cognition, 31, 34–37, 52, 62, 110
  development of, 11–12, 55, 65, 75–79
  distinctions among negative, 80–82
  effects of unbearable, 138, 140
  incapacity for, 4–5, 24, 34
  and intention, 9–11, 34–37
  and memory, 61–62, 132–133
  role of, 11–12, 76
  in Russell's theories, 72–73, 118
  in therapeutic relationship, 133–136
  therapist sharing patient's, 26–27, 53–54, 140–141
  therapist's resistance to feeling patient's, 18–19, 25
  in Tomkins's theories, 73–76, 105–106
  transformation of, 6, 43–44

Affect, Imagery, Consciousness (Tomkins), 74, 82
Affect categories, 61–64
Affect regulation, 62–63, 65
  of infants, 78–79
  mutual, 63, 137
Affect training, 62–65
Affective competence, 38. *See also* Affective incompetence
  growth of, 11–12, 64–65, 115–116
  and relationships, 9–10, 37
Affective exchange, between therapist and patient, 53–54
Affective incompetence, 113
  repetition compulsion as, 7–9, 61, 123, 125
Aggression, 10, 25
  and death instinct, 42–43
  defenses against, 116–117
American Psychological Association, local chapters movement of, 49
Amplification of affect, 76, 78, 88, 106
Anger
  at pain of repetition compulsion, 9
  in Tomkins's script theories, 86, 95–96, 98

INDEX

Anger (*continued*)
 in Tomkins's theories of discrete affects, 81–82
Anscombe, R., 19, 31
Antinomy, and paradox, 109–110
Anti-toxic script, 95–100
Anxiety, role of, 11
Attachment, 11, 44
 effects of, 20, 36–37
 ruptures of, 27–28, 90, 125–126, 130–132, 134, 137, 140
 in therapeutic relationship, 16–17, 20, 54, 124, 137
Atwood, G., 138

Basch, M. F., 73
Bergmann, M., 141
Beyond the Pleasure Principle (Freud), 41, 87, 128
"Beyond the Wish" (Russell), 24
Bibring, E., 11
Bion, W. R., 89
Bodily processes
 changes from affects, 11, 74–75
 trauma and healing, 32–33
Bowlby, J., 127, 130
Breuer, J., 39–40
Bromberg, P. M., 51–52
Buffalo Creek disaster, 27–29

Cannon, W. B., 32–33
Caregivers
 in decontamination script, 92–93
 and infants' affect, 76–79, 137
 recreating relationship with therapist, 134
Change, *vs.* continuity, 51–52, 57

Cognition, 56
 and action, 34–37
 relation to affect, 11, 31, 34–37, 52, 110
 relation to memory, 61–62
Coherence, *vs.* completeness, 21
Competence, *vs.* repetition, 4–6
Complemental series of traumata, 39–40
Completeness, *vs.* consistency, 15–16, 21, 110
Containment, 46, 67–68
 need for, 38–39
 process of, 27–28
 Russell's gift for, 106–108, 115
 in treatment, 19–20, 24, 117
 of wishes, 10, 25, 44–45, 53–54
Continuity, *vs.* change, 51–52, 57
Control, and guilt after rape, 28–29
Countertransference, 133
 resistance to, 17, 141
Cowardice, in decontamination script, 91–92

Death instinct, 41–44
 as explanation for repetition compulsion, 60, 87, 128–129
Decontamination script, 85–86
 disgust in, 90–93
 vs. anti-toxic, 99–101
Defenses, 97–99, 116–117
Depression, 11, 37–38
Development, 10, 55–56, 119, 127, 130
 affective, 11–12, 55, 63, 65, 75–79
 of personality, 83–84

148

INDEX

Disgust, 81
  in decontamination script, 85–86, 90–93, 99
Distress, in Tomkins's theories, 80–81, 85
Dysfunction, as sign of injury, 34

Edelman, G., 61–62
Ekman, P., 73
Empathy, for patient, 30–31, 52
Erikson, K., 27–29

Fairbairn, R. W. D., 51, 54
Fantasy, vs. reality, 40
Fear
  in Tomkins's script theories, 86, 95–96, 98
  in Tomkins's theories of discrete affects, 80–82
"Fear of Breakdown, The" (Winnicott), 134
Feelings. See Affect
Fishman, G., 3, 141
Frank, A., 73
Freud, S., 9–11, 25
  on affect, 9–10, 74, 76
  on components of trauma, 39–42
  on repetition compulsion, 1–2, 8, 51, 60, 86–88
  Russell's use of, 51, 126–127, 128–129
Friedman, L., 54
Friesen, W. V., 73

Ghent, E., 54–55
Gödel, K., 15, 108, 110, 112

Grandiosity, in decontamination script, 91–95
Greed, in decontamination script, 91–92
Greenberg, J., 52
Grief, 133, 139
  and repetition compulsion, 9, 124–125
Guilt, in rape trauma, 28–29

Haley, S., 26–27
Hate, 45
  relation to love, 43–44
  in therapeutic relationship, 133–134
Healing
  physical and psychic, 32–33, 69–71
  requirements for, 2–3, 67–68, 116, 142
Herman, J., 127, 140
Herzog, J., 141
Holocaust, dealing with trauma of, 141
Hypervigilance, in Tomkins's anti-toxic script, 97

Ideo–affect complexes, 75–76
Infants. See also Development
  affects of, 73–79
  and mutual affect regulation, 63, 137
Inhibition, 10
Injury. See also Trauma
  and gaining affective competence, 115–116
  physical models for psychic, 69–71

INDEX

Intention. *See also* Wishes
  and affect, 9–11
  and psychic trauma, 128–129
  and requirements for healing, 116
Internalization, and transference repetition, 131
Interpersonal psychoanalysis, 72–73, 76
Interpretations, 54, 136–137
Intersubjectivists, 127, 137–139
Intrapsychic processes, *vs.* interpersonal, 73, 76–77, 79
Introjects, incompleteness of, 108, 112
Izard, C., 73

Kant, I., 118
Kernberg, O., 39
Klein, M., 11, 39
Kohut, H., 10
Kuhn, T. S., 13, 51, 108, 110

Lacan, J., 113
Lakoff, G., 61
Learning, and compulsion to repeat, 4–6
Levenson, on repetition compulsion, 51
Lindy, J. D., 99
Loewald, E., 131
Loewald, H., 51, 60
  compared to Russell, 117, 127
  compared to Winnicott, 56–57
  on perpetual tensions, 55–57
  on transference repetition, 130–133

Loneliness, 27, 35
  in Tomkins's script theories, 97–100
Love
  capacity for, 45–46
  relation to hate, 43–44

Magnification of affect, 82–83, 88
  in Tomkins's script theories, 82–83, 96–97
Malatesta, C., 86–89
Masochism, and repetition compulsion, 23–24
Mastery
  of affect, 39
  repetition compulsion as attempt at, 4, 23, 89–90
Mazer, H., 140
McCombie, S., 28
Memory, 61, 111
  advances in field, 61–62
  and mourning, 132–133
  and past and present, 28–29, 135
  and repetition, 3–4
  and repetition compulsion, 24, 123
Metaphors
  in memory theories, 61–62
  in psychoanalysis, 64, 117
Metonymic associations, 61–62, 64
Mitchell, S. A., 57
Mitrani, J. L., 89
Modell, A., 127
  on affect, 11, 61–62
  on therapeutic relationship, 134–136

INDEX

Mothers. *See also* Caregivers
   in affective development, 63, 65
Mourning, and memory, 132–133
Mutual affect regulation, 63, 137

Nagel, E., 15
Nathanson, D. L., 73
Negotiation
   and affective competence, 9–10, 19, 133–134
   in therapeutic relationship, 16–18, 112–116, 133–134, 138
   and transference, 9, 19–20
Neurosis, from repression, 10
Newman, J. R., 15

Objectivity, relation to thoughts and feelings, 36
"On the Therapeutic Action of Psychoanalysis" (Loewald), 130
Other Times, Other Realities (Modell), 135

Pain
   role in injury and healing, 33–34
   as species of hate, 43
Paradox, 15–16, 60, 94
   and antinomy, 109–110
   negotiation of, 113–116
   in Russell's theories, 54–58, 108–114
   of transference, 19–20
   usefulness for growth, 12–15, 20–21, 57–58
   in Winnicott's theories, 133

Paranoia, 30–31, 37–38
Parents. *See* Caregivers; Mothers
Past *vs.* present, 135–136
   differentiation of, 113, 132
   influence of past traumas, 60, 141
   in psychoanalytic theory, 59–60
Pearlman, L. A., 99
Perception, and memory, 111
Personality, 83–86
Pizer, S., 54, 112
Poverty, trauma of, 29
Present. *See* Past *vs.* present
Primary *vs.* secondary processes, 55–56, 57
Principia Mathematica (Russell and Whitehead), 14
Projective identification, 39, 116–117
Psychoanalysis, 64, 119
   changing attitudes in, 59–60, 112
   Russell in range of theories of, 126–142
Psychopathology, 52
   and repetition compulsion, 24, 51
Psychosis, 8, 140

Quine, W. V., 108–109

Rage. *See* Anger
Rako, S., 139
Rape, trauma from, 28–29
Reality, 25, 38
   and feelings, 35–37, 45–46
   and trauma, 26–29, 40

INDEX

Relational psychoanalysis. *See* Interpersonal psychoanalysis
Relationships
   containment of wishes in, 25, 44–45
   continuation of, 16–17, 44–45, 114, 138, 140
   continuity supplied through, 52
   functions of, 19, 29–31, 36–37, 72–73, 125–126
   and repetition compulsion, 4, 7–8
"Remembering, Repeating, and Working Through" (Freud), 128
Renik, O., 141
Repetition, 12
   purposes of, 1, 4–5
   in therapeutic relationship, 136–137
Repetition compulsion, 9, 20
   as affective incompetence, 35, 123, 125
   death instinct as explanation for, 60, 128–129
   explanations for, 7, 39, 51, 62, 120, 130–132
   Freud's explanations for, 41–42, 86–88
   purposes of, 1–4
   Russell's explanations for, 61, 126
   and self-fulfilling prophecies, 135–136
   in therapeutic relationship, 41, 64, 113–116
   and trauma, 23–24
   vs. decontamination script theory, 86, 90–91
Repression, as method of control, 10
Resistance, 134
   and repetition compulsion, 2, 6–8
   therapist's, 17–19, 53, 139–140
"Role of Paradox in Affect and the Repetition Compulsion, The" (Russell), 59–60
Rorty, R., 108
Russell, B., 14
Russell, P.
   on affect training, 62–65
   explanations for repetition compulsion, 87, 89–90, 125
   influence of, 49–50, 59
   place in psychoanalytic range, 126–142
   on psychoanalysis, 117–118, 124
   on relationships, 72–73
   as supervisor, 106–108, 114–115
   on trauma, 65, 69–72
   on treatment crises, 52, 113–114, 142–143
   use of paradox theories, 54–58
   writings of, 50–51

Saakvitne, K. W., 99
Santayana, G., 4
Schore, A. N., 63, 137
Script theory, Tomkins's, 82–86
Sedgewick, E. K., 73
Seduction, in decontamination script, 91–93, 95

INDEX

Self
  fear of disintegration, 63
  sense of, 10, 113
Self-fulfilling prophecies, 135–136
Semrad, E., 127, 139–140
Sexuality, 40, 43
  intention and affect in, 9–10, 25
Shame, in Tomkins's theories, 80, 85
Sifneos, P., 32
Smith, B., 84
Smith, L. B., 62, 119
Social fabric, damage to, 28
Spezzano, C., 52
Splitting, 39
Stern, D. N., 63, 89, 119, 137
Stoller, R. J., 43
Stolorow, R., 137–139
Structure of Scientific Revolutions, The (Kuhn), 13
Suicide, 8
Symptoms, in Tompkins's scripts, 99–100

Terror. *See* Fear
Thelen, E., 62, 119
"Theory of the Crunch, The" (Russell), 24
Therapist, 99, 123–124. *See also* Transference
  containment by, 67–68, 117
  patient's view of, 94–95
  relationship with patients, 16–17, 131–132
  repetitions by, 30–31, 126
  resistance of, 17–19, 53, 139–140
  role of, 52–53, 136–137
  sharing patient's feelings, 26, 53–54, 113–114, 140–142
  theories of, 68–69
Tomkins, S., 105
  script theories of, 82–86, 90–93, 95–100
  theories of affects of, 73–76, 80–82
Transference, 54, 94
  and repetition compulsion, 4, 41, 88
  risks of, 8–9
  role in treatment, 16–17, 19–20
  Russell's explanations for, 52–53
Transference repetition, 64, 130–133
Transitional space, 133, 135
Trauma, 26, 43–44, 99
  causes of, 9, 25, 70–71, 138
  components of, 39–41
  effects of, 7, 26–31, 140
  repetition of, 2–4, 8, 20, 23–24
  role in Russell's theories, 65, 72, 127–130
  vs. Tomkins's anti-toxic script, 95–100
  wishes and reality in, 26–27
"Trauma and the Cognitive Function of Affect" (Russell), 61
Treatment, 133
  crises in, 15–19, 24, 29–31, 52–53, 123, 125–126, 137, 142–143
  goals of, 65, 117
  methods of, 45–46, 113–114, 138–139, 142

INDEX

Treatment (*continued*)
   and paradoxes of transference, 19–20
   patient's scripts in, 94–95, 97–98
   repetition in, 26, 41
   risks of, 8–9
Tronick, E., 65
Trust, in therapeutic relationships, 29–31, 54

Urgencies, 9, 10
   grief as, 125–126
   therapist's, 18, 52–53

Validity, relation to thought and feeling, 35
van der Kolk, B., 127, 140
Vietnam War veterans, trauma of, 26–27
Vulnerability, as result of painful affects, 71

Whitehead, A. N., 14
Wilson, A., 86–89
Wilson, J. P., 99
Winnicott, D. W., 51, 56, 113
   compared to Loewald, 56–57
   compared to Russell, 127
   on hate, 42–43
   on therapeutic relationship, 133–134
Wishes, 35. *See also* Intention
   capacity for, 24–25
   and death instinct, 41–44
   and preservation of relationships, 44, 52–53
   in repetition compulsion, 89, 123
   transformation of, 43–44
   and trauma, 26–29, 40, 128–129
Wittgenstein, L., 108

Zetzel, E., 11, 37–38

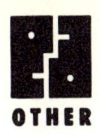

Also of interest from The Other Press...

Before I Was I: Psychoanalysis and the Imagination
Enid Balint (ed.)

Wilfred Bion: His Life and Works 1897–1979
Gerard Bleandonu

Slouching Towards Bethlehem
Nina Coltart

The Clinical Lacan
Joël Dor

Introduction to the Reading of Lacan
Joël Dor

Fairbairn and the Origins of Object Relations
James S. Grotstein and Donald B. Rinsley (eds.)

*Lacan and the New Wave in American Psychoanalysis:
The Subject and the Self*
Judith Feher Gurewich and Michel Tort (eds.)

Motherhood and Sexuality
Marie Langer

Lacanian Psychotherapy with Children: The Broken Piano
Catherine Mathelin

Hysteria from Freud to Lacan: The Splendid Child of Psychoanalysis
Juan-David Nasio

Mother, Madonna, Whore: The Idealization and Denigration of Motherhood
Estella V. Welldon

Hierarchical Concepts in Psychoanalysis
Arnold Wilson and John E. Gedo (eds.)

www.otherpress.com   toll free 877-THE OTHER (843-6843)